A

SHORT ACCOUNT

OF THE

MATERIA MEDICA OF PATNA

BY

R. H. IRVINE

GYAN

Published by

Gyan Publishing House
5, Ansari Road
Daryaganj, New Delhi-110002
Phone: 011-47034999, 9811692060
E-mail: books@gyanbooks.com

Distribution Network
gyanbooks.com
India, USA, Canada, UK, Australia

ISBN: 978-93-6433-339-9 (PB)
First Published, 1848

2nd Impression 2024

Printed at: Gyan Press, Delhi.

A SHORT ACCOUNT OF THE MATERIA MEDICA OF PATNA
Author: R. H. IRVINE

A

SHORT ACCOUNT

OF THE

MATERIA MEDICA OF PATNA

A SHORT ACCOUNT OF THE MATERIA MEDICA OF PATNA.

BY R. H. IRVINE, M. D.,
CIVIL SURGEON.

PRINTED BY ORDER OF GOVERNMENT.

CALCUTTA:
W. RIDSDALE, MILITARY ORPHAN PRESS.
1848.

SHORT ACCOUNT

Here also, almost every wealthy inhabitant becomes impotent or in a state tending to that from excessive early dissipation, and as such, people will pay well for relief, a great number of substances are employed in a very preposterous manner with the view of benefitting in that way, hence a large part of the Patna Pharmacopœia, consists of substances employed for their supposed aphrodisial virtues.

Nearly all the articles of real efficacy used by the Natives are found in our own Pharmacopœia, such as gamboge, impure calomel, pure corrosive sublimate, arsenious acid, senna, cassia fistula, sulphur, mercury, opium, musk, castor, croton tiglium, rhubarb, turbeth root, jalap, impure potash and soda, the impure mineral acids, and several others.

The general nature of their prescriptions is ridiculous in regard to combination and quality of materials.

Such, however, as are the numerous substances sold by the punsaries or native apothecaries, still, though generally very cheap and easily procured, they are constantly adulterated, being under no regulation and liable to no investigation whatever; they are at liberty to injure the lieges of the Hon'ble Company, to a full extent, and especially the quantity of arsenic and other poisons sold is terrible to think of.

The latter evil might be greatly obviated by placing all the punsaries under certain proper restrictions; compelling such to bring a written list with small accompanying specimens, twice a year, to the Civil Surgeon for inspection; and levying a fine where the articles were not genuine; and by compelling punsaries to bring a written account of all the worst kinds of poisons sold, with the names and residences of the purchasers, once a month, to the Magistrate. At least, at Civil and Military stations, something of this kind might be effected.

I now subjoin the four hundred and eighty articles of any consequence as medicines, selected from the Patna Native apothecaries.

This account of the Patna Native Materia Medica was drawn up to accompany a box containing the 480 specimens of every article described, and carefully arranged for reference when desired.

In all cases the native opinion regarding the action and doses of these remedies has been entered. Some of the articles are ridiculous in application or nearly inert; while many are efficacious, and in the hands of the superior hukeems are applied in reference to qualities nearly in accordance with modern scientific views.

These articles were selected from the "punsaries'" shops at Patna, and, comprise all that possess any energy, per se, or implied efficacy by collateral influence of magic.

In relation to the general state of the native practice of physic, the higher Hindoo castes act the most wisely in rejecting interference altogether, and holding with Pliny, that "omnis morbus lethalis aut curabilis; in vitam desinit aut in mortem. Utroque igitur modo medicina inutilis; si lethalis, curari non potest; si curabilis, non requirit medicum; natura expellat;" and they live or die resigned and contented.

But by far the greater number of sick are a prey to native "mountebanks, empirics, quacksalvers or wizards, barbers, and old women."

Quibus loquacis affatim arrogantiæ est,
Peritiæ parum aut nihil!

The community having full faith in the Paracelsian adage, that relief depends not so much on remedial action as upon psychological imbuement through the medium of the preparer; so that with them

Hellebrorus curat; sed quod ab omni datus medico, vanum est!

The native surgery of Patna is at a still lower ebb than the native physic; and of both of the most numerous and inferior order of professors it may be truly said—

Chirurgus medico quo differt? scilicetisto,
Enecat *hic* succis; enecat *ille* manu.

Names, English and Country.	Botanical Names.	Remarks.
No. 1. Asgandh, Isgandh. Ashwaragandha. आश्वगंध اسگندھ	Physalis. Flexuosa.	The root used in substance and decoction as diuretic and deobstruent. Dose from ℈ss. to ʒi. in powder. Price per lb. 0 3 4
No. 2. Amahuldi. Amada. Mangoe Ginger. आमाहलदी اماهلدي	Curcuma. Amada.	The root used as carminative and to promote digestion. Dose from ℈i. to ʒii. Price per lb. 0 1 8
No. 3. Anisun. आनीशुष انيسون	Pimpinella. Anisun.	Imported and used as carminative and to promote digestion. The seed— Dose from ℈i. to ʒii. Price per lb. 0 5 0
No. 4. Agusti. Agati Grandiflora. Œschynomene Grandiflora. आगस्तः اگست	Agati Grandiflora. Œschynomene. Grandiflora.	The bark used in infusion as febrifuge. Dose ℥ii. of the infusion. Price per lb. 0 2 0

Names, English and Country.	Botanical Names.	Remarks.
No. 5. Akurkurra. Indian Pellitory. आकरकारः عقرقرہ	Anthemis. Pyrethrum.	The root imported and used as an external as well as internal stimulant and sialagogue. Dose from ℈i. to ʒi. Price per lb. 0 12 0
No. 6. Asaroon. Asara Bacca. आसारया اسارون	Asarum Europœum.	The dry plant imported from Persia, used as a stimulant. Dose ℈i. Price per lb. 0 4 0
No. 7. Arusa. Bakus. आरुष اروس اروسا	Justicia Adhatoda. Adhatoda Vasica.	Common every where, root used in decoction, in colds, and fevers. Dose from ℥ss. to ℥i. of the decoction. Price per lb. 0 1 0
No. 8. Ajowain. आजवैया اجواين	Ligusticum. Ajowan.	Cultivated, seed used as carminative and to promote digestion, used also externally. Dose from ʒss. to ʒi. Price per lb. 0 0 8

Names, English and Country.	Botanical Names.	Remarks.
No. 9. Ajmod. Indian Parsley. आजमोदः اجموده	Apium. Involucratum.	Cultivated, the seed used as carminative and diuretic and to promote digestion. Dose from ʒss. to ʒi. Price per lb. 0 0 8
No. 10. Apheem. Opium. आफीम افيون	Papaver Somniferum.	Immensely cultivated and exported. Largely used as a sedative and stimulant, both for intoxication and medicinally, internally and externally. Dose from gr. i. to gr. iii. Price per lb. 5 0 0
No. 11. Ajmod Khorasanee. आजमोद खोराशानी اجموده خراساني	Œnanthe. Phellandrium.	The seed imported from Persia, and given in colds. Dose from gr. v. to ℈ss. Price per lb. 0 3 0
No. 12. Ajowan Khorasanee. Henbane. आजोवान खोराशानी اجواين خراساني	Hyosciamus Niger.	The seed imported largely, used in food as carminative and stimulant, also in medicine. Dose from gr. v. to ℈ss. Price per lb. 0 2 0

Names, English and Country.	Botanical Names.	Remarks.
No. 13. Amultas Kaphull. अमलतास का फल املتاس	Catharto—carpus. Fistula. Cassia Fistula.	The pulp of the pods much used as a laxative; the tree very common and beautiful. Dose from ʒii. to ℥ss. Price per lb. 0 2 0
No. 14. Anoola, Anola. آنوله	Emblica Officinalis. Phyllanthus. Emblica.	The fruit much used as a dye, also internally as a pickle, and dried as an astringent. I have given it copiously in scurvy, with benefit. Dose from ℥ss. to ℥i. Price per lb. 0 0 8
No. 15. Aritha. Ritha. रीठा ریٹھا	Sapindus Detergens.	The fruit much used in dyeing, also applied externally as discutient. Dose gandum sufficit. Price per lb. 0 0 8
No. 16. Ach. Al. आछ اچهه	Morinda Tinctoria and Citrifolia.	The root much used in dyeing, also given internally as astringent. Dose from ℈i. to ʒi. of the bark of the root. Price per lb. 0 2 0

Names, English and Country.	Botanical Names.	Remarks.
No. 17. Abrakh. आबरख ابرکهہ		Mica and talc, used burnt in fevers. Dose from ʒi. to ʒss. Price per lb. 0 2 0
No. 18. Akakiya. आकाकीया اقاقيا	Acacia Vera.	A red extract of the wood, used as a powerful astringent. Dose from ʒi. to ʒii. Price per lb. 5 8 0
No. 19. Aphtemun. Amr-bel. Indian Dodder. आफतीमुन افتيمون	Cuscuta Reflexa.	Common on many trees, used externally as discutient, considered a charm. Dose from gr. v. to ʒi. Price per lb. 0 0 2
No. 20. Aphtemun Wilayte. आफतीमुन वीलायती Dodder Wormwood. افتيمون ولايتي	Cuscuta Reflexa.	The dried leaves imported from Bombay, used as discutient externally, internally as cathartic and emetic. Dose from gr. ii. to gr. v. Price per lb. 4 0 0

Names, English and Country.	Botanical Names.	Remarks.
No. 21. Akut. Choonie. आकुत ياقوت چني		Small garnets, used pounded up as an aphrodisiac; small rubies also used in the same way. Dose ℈i. to ʒi. Price per lb. 45 0 0
No. 22. Aprung. Rung Bhurrut. Dum-ul Ukhwain. Heera Dukhan. आपरंग دم الاخوين	Calamus Draco. Pterocarpus Draco.	A kind of dragon's blood brought from Bombay, and used as an astringent. This is generally from the Calamus Draco, and is a very fine kind. Dose ʒi. to ʒiii. Price per lb. 17 10 0
No. 23. Abresham. आबरेशम ابريشم		White silk, cut up very fine and used as an aphrodisiac. Dose ℈ss. Price per lb. 6 0 0

Names, English and Country.	Botanical Names.	Remarks.
No. 24. Ak, Mudar. Madar. आक آک	Calotropis Gigantea. Asclepias Gigantea.	The root is used, the bark being pounded, it is similar to ipecacuanha, but more uncertain, it is excellent in leprosy; the down and juice are applied externally in many cases. Dose gr. v. to ʒi. Price per lb. 0 0 8
No. 25. Amber. Ambergris. अमबर عنبر		Brought from Singapore, used as aphrodisiac. Dose gr. v. to ℈ss. Price per lb. 80 0 0
No. 26. Bhee Dana. भीदाना بيهي دانه	Cydonia Vulgaris.	Common quince seed, used as demulcent in sherbets, imported from Cabul. Dose ʒii. to ℥i. Price per lb. 2 2 0
No. 27. Bekh-bunufsha. Orris Root. बेखबनफ्शः بيخ بنفشه	Iris Florentina.	Imported from Cabul, used as a scent and stimulant. Dose gr. v. to ℈i. Price per lb. 1 0 0

Names, English and Country.	Botanical Names.	Remarks.
No. 28. Bekh-kurphus. Spikenard Roots. वेखकरपस بیخ کرفس	Nardostachys Jatamansi.	Used as a stimulant, and in scents, imported from Nepal. There are several kinds, of which this is the best. Dose gr. v. to ℈i. Price per lb. 6 0 0
No. 29. Badam, sweet Almonds. बादाम بادام	Amygdalus Communis.	Used as restorative and aphrodisiac. Dose ℥ii. to lb. i. Price per lb. 0 4 0
No. 30. Bol-i-armanie. Armenian Bole. बोलआरमनी بورهٔ ارمني		Used as an astringent; and eaten at times, and applied to sores. Dose ℈i. to ʒi. Price per lb. 5 3 0
No. 31. Burmie. Bhirmie Sugandh. Ewe Tree. भीरमीसुगंधः برمي سوگنده	Taxus Baccata.	Used in scent and as an aphrodisiac. Dose gr. ii. Price per lb. 5 0 0

Names, English and Country.	Botanical Names.	Remarks.
No. 32. Bhoji-dan. भोजीदाना بوزیدان	Colchicum Byzantinum.	A white root, brought from Cabul, considered stimulant, and used as an aphrodisiac. Dose gr. ss. to gr. iss. Price per lb. 0 1 0
No. 33. Bhaboona Soorookh. Camomile Root. बाबुनासुरख بهمن سرخ	Anthemis Nobilis.	Brought from the N. W. P., used as tonic and febrifuge. Dose ℈i. to ʒii. Price per lb. 3 0 0
No. 34. Bhaboona Sufaid. बाबुनासफेद بهمن سفید	Anthemis Arvensis.	Field camomile, used as a tonic and febrifuge. Dose ℈i. to ʒii. Price per lb. 3 0 0
No. 35. Bunafsha. Sweet Violet. बनफशः بنفشه	Viola Odorifera.	The whole plant comes dried from the hills, used in fevers, as heating and stimulant and sudorific; also as an emetic to children. Dose ℈i. to ℈ii. Price per lb. 6 0 0

Names, English and Country.	Botanical Names.	Remarks.
No. 36. Bunafsha Mugrabi. बनफशामगरबी بنفشه مغربي	Egyptian Violets.	Imported; used as heating and stimulant; and sudorific. Dose gr. v. to ℈i. Price per lb. 5 0 0
No. 37. Bartung. Rib Grass. बारतंग بارتنگ	Plantago Lanceolata.	An angular glassy seed imported; used as cooling and astringent; given in sherbets in diarrhœa. Dose ʒii. to ℥i. Price per lb. 0 8 0
No. 38. Bol. Myrrh. बोल بول	Balsamo dendron Myrrha.	Also in India from the amyris agallocha (plentiful about Ajmeer,) used internally as stimulant; and to wounds. Dose gr. ii. to ℈ss. Price per lb. 3 0 0
No. 39. Banslochun. Tabasheer. बंसलोचन بنس لوچن	Bambusa Arundinacea.	Silicious concrete found in bamboos; used as an aphrodisiac; and in charms. Dose gr. v. to ℈i. Price per lb. 48 0 0

Names, English and Country.	Botanical Names.	Remarks.
No. 40. Burg-furing-mushk. बगफरंजमुश्क برگ فرنج مشک	Dorema Ammoniacum.	Scented leaves, imported, used as stimulants. The dried leaves of the gum ammoniac plant. Dose ℈i. to ʒss. Price per lb. 18 0 0
No. 41. Bisfayaz. Common Polypody. बीस्फेयाज بصفياغ	Polypodium Vulgare.	Roots imported from the Hills, used as a stimulant; given in flatulent indigestion. Dose gr. v. to ℈i. Price per lb. 1 8 6
No. 42. Boondee. बुन्दी بوندي		Mixture of lead and zinc, used externally to sores. Dose in ointments ʒi. per ℥i. Ungt. Price per lb. 0 2 6
No. 43. Bhadiyan Kutai. बादीयाखताई باديان خطائي	Illicium Anisatum.	Seed and pods used as carminative and stimulant. Dose gr. x. to ℈ii. Price per lb. 6 0 0

Names, English and Country.	Botanical Names.	Remarks.
No. 44. Bekh-unjubaz. बेखश्रानजुबाज् بیخ انجوباز	Polygonum Barbatum.	Root imported from the N. W. P., used as cooling and astringent. Dose gr. v. to ℈i. Price per lb. 3 0 0
No. 45. Bukam. Indian Brazil Wood. बकम بکم	Cœsalpinia Sappan.	Used in dyeing; and as an astringent in medicines. Also called pattung. Dose ℈i. to ʒii. Price per lb. 0 1 0
No. 46. Bha-khoomba. बाखुमबा باکھومبہ	Trichosanthes Cordata.	Dried flowers, used as a stimulant. Dose gr. ii. to gr. v. Price per lb. 1 8 0
No. 47. Bhilawan. Marking Nut. भीलावाबा بھلاوان	Semicarpus Anacardium.	Fruit eaten when given. Juice of dry nut, very acrid and used as an escharotic; and much more painful than Cantharides; given internally in syphilis. Dose gr. ss. to ℈i. Price per lb. 0 1 8

Names, English and Country.	Botanical Names.	Remarks.
No. 48. Bhai-birrung. बाबिरंग بابرنگ	Embelia Ribes.	Dried fruit, brought from the Hills; used as heating and stimulant. Dose gr. v. to ℈ii. Price per lb. 0 1 8
No. 49. Bhurungi. भरंगी بهارنگي	Nima Quassioides.	Bark brought from the Hills; used as heating and stimulant. Dose gr. v. to ʒi. Price per lb. 0 1 9
No. 50. Bhij-bund. बीजबंद Tripakshi. بيجبند	Coldenia Procumbeus.	Small shining angular seeds, brought from the N. W. P., used as an aphrodisiac; also common in the rice fields at Patna. Dose ℈i. to ʒii. Price per lb. 0 1 8
No. 51. Badaward. Called also Shookai. बादश्रावरद باداورد	Cacalia Sonchifolia.	Twigs, leaves and flowers, brought from the Hills; used as stimulant and expectorant. Dose ℈ii. to ʒiii. Price per lb. 6 0 0

Names, English and Country.	Botanical Names.	Remarks.
No. 52. Birrun-ja-sif. Mugwort. बीरञ्जासीफ برنج آسف	Artemisia Vulgaris.	Used as a valuable bitter stomachic; also in infusion as deobstruent and antispasmodic. The dried leaves and flowers come from the Hills. Dose ℈ss. to ʒi. Price per lb. 6 0 0
No. 53. Bahira. Belleric Myrobalan. बाहीरा بهيرا	Terminialia Bellerica.	Fruit and seed used in dyeing; and as a laxative and astringent. Dose gr. v. to ℈ii. Price per lb. 0 0 8
No. 54. Balchur. Called also Ooshur. बालछर بالچهر	Valeriana Hardwickii. (?)	Root of a species of nardostachys, imported from the Hills; used in vast quantities to scent and clean the hair. This is by far the most common kind; and is also given in medicine as refreshment. Dose gr. v. to ʒi. Price per lb. 0 2 0

Names, English and Country.	Botanical Names.	Remarks.
No. 55. Burg-sudab. Caper Euphorbium. बरगशुदाब برگ سداب	Euphorbia Lathyris.	Imported dried leaves, fruits and stalks, used as a carminative in Dyspepsia; and as deobstruent. Dose gr. i. to gr. iii. Price per lb. 0 8 0
No. 56. Bel-ka-putta. बेल का पत्ता بیل کا پته	Cratœva Marmelos. Œgle Marmelos.	Leaves used in enchantments; and given in fevers; fruit much used in dysentery and diarrhœa. Dose ℥i. to ℥ii. Price per lb. 0 0 6
No. 57. Badrung-boya. बादरंजबोया بادرنج بویا	Melissa Repens.	The whole plant brought from Nepal, used as carminative and as a scent. Dose gr. v. to ʒss. Price per lb. 0 8 0
No. 58. Babai. Lemon Toolsee. बाबै بابئي	Ocimum Pilosum.	The whole plant delightfully fragrant; the seeds used as demulcent and refrigerant. The whole plant smells like verbena. Dose ℥ss. Price per lb. 0 0 8

Names, English and Country.	Botanical Names.	Remarks.
No. 59. Bhikma. भीखमा بهیکهمه	Aconitum Heterophyllum.	The root imported from Nepal; bitter, hot and poisonous; is given in ghee to cure colic; and as aphrodisiac. Dose gr. ss. to gr. i. Price per lb. 0 6 0
No. 60. Bishnag. Vishnaga. बीशनाग بش ناک	Aconitum Ferox.	The root brought from Nepal, called " meethazahur," and much used in poisoning; also used to poison arrows; and as aphrodisiac. Dose gr. $\frac{1}{16}$ Price per lb. 6 12 0
No. 61. Cheraytta. चेरेता چریتا	Agathotes Cheraytta.	The whole dried plant brought from Nepal; there are two species, one of which is very narcotic; the common kind is universally used as an excellent tonic. Dose ʒss. in infusion. Price per lb. 0 8 0

Names, English and Country.	Botanical Names.	Remarks.
No. 62. Cabob Cheny. कबाबचीनी كباب چيني	Piper Cubeba.	Cubebs, used as cooling and diuretic; also in food. Dose ℈i. to ʒiii. Price per lb. 0 6 0
No. 63. Choonee Gond. चुनीगोंद چنيا گوند	Butea Frondosa.	Indian kino; used as an excellent astringent. Dose ʒss. to ʒii. Price per lb. 0 3 0
No. 64. Chundun Safaid. चनदण सफेद چندن سفيد	Santalum Album.	Sandal-wood, used as a scent; and cooling carminative. Dose ʒss. to ʒi. Price per lb. 0 4 0
No. 65. Chundun Lall. Also Rukht Chundun. Red Saunders Wood. चनदण लाल چندن سرخ	Pterocarpus Santalinus.	Used in dyeing; also as astringent and cooling. Dose ʒss. to ʒi. Price per lb. 0 4 0

Names, English and Country.	Botanical Names.	Remarks.
No. 66. Chob Chinee. चोबचीनी Shookh Chinee. چوب چيني	Smilax Chinensis.	The root imported from China and Rungpore, used in decoction as highly restorative; often adulterated with the old roots of Tagetes Erecta. Dose ʒii. to ℥i. Price per lb. 0 14 0
No. 67. Chironjee. चीरोंजी چيرونجي	Buchanania Latifolia.	The seeds are called Chironjee and used as Almonds; the fruit called "achar," "आक्कार:" is eaten raw. Dose ℥i. to ℥ii. Price per lb. 0 8 0
No. 68. Chook-ka-beej. चुक का बीच چوک کا بيج	Rumex Vesicaria.	Seed of the bladder sorrel; cooling and astringent. Dose ℈i. to ʒss. Price per lb. 0 0 8
No. 69. Chohara. छोहारा چھوهاره	Phœnix Dactylifera.	Dates imported dry and moist; restorative. Dose ℥i. to ℥iii. Price per lb. 0 3 0

Names, English and Country.	Botanical Names.	Remarks.
No. 70. Chitruk Lall. चीतरक लाल Red Lead Wort. لال چتا چترکهه لال	Plumbago Rosea.	The root sialagogne; and vesicatory; and stimulant. Dose gr. ss. to gr. iii. Price per lb. 1 2 0
No. 71. Chitruk Sufaid. White Lead Wort. चीतरक सफेद چترکهه سفید	Plumbago Zeylanica.	The root sialagogne; and vesicatory; and stimulant. Dose gr. ss. to gr. iii. Price per lb. 0 0 8
No. 72. Churrus. चरस Extract of Indian Hemp. چرس	Cannabis Indica.	This is both a resinous exudation; as well as an artificial preparation, and largely used as a general narcotic stimulant and aphrodisiac. The best is extracted by men in leather aprons, running through the fields of the wild plant when the resinous exudation adheres and is scraped off and kept as very superior. The worst is made by boiling the whole plant. Dose gr. ¼ to ℈i. Price per lb. 96 0 0

Names, English and Country.	Botanical Names.	Remarks.
No. 73. Choka. चोका چوکهه	Convolvulus Bryonifolius.	Root brought from Cabul, used to cure the itch; externally applied in diseases of Camels; and taken internally as narcotic. Dose gr. ss. Price per lb. 0 6 0
No. 74. Chumpontie. Clubbed Dendrobium. चमपौटी چنپوتي	Dendrobium Clavatum.	The dried plant comes from Nepal; used in scent; and as an aphrodisiœ. Dose ℈i. to ʒii. Price per lb. 5 0 0
No. 75. Chakowar. चोकोवार Junglee Powar. چکوره	Cassia Obtusifolia.	Jungli pooar. The seed taken whole to cleanse the blood. Dose gr. v. to ℈ss. Price per lb. 0 1 0

Names, English and Country.	Botanical Names.	Remarks.
No. 76. Chak ; Chook. चुक چوک	Rumex Vesicaria.	An extract used as cooling in sherbets. Dose ℈i. to ʒii. Price per lb. 0 6 0
No. 77. Chumbranak. चमवरानक چمرانکهه		Valve of a shell fish; as "sitanuk" "शीटानकः" is the fish and valve united; imported from Calcutta; and used as aphrodisiac. Dose ʒii. to ℥ss. Price per lb. 7 8 0
No. 78. Cajuputte-ka-tel. Ilachie-ka-tel. इलाची का तेल الايچي کا تيل	Melaleuca Leucadendron.	Imported and used as carminative and stimulant; also rubefacient. Dose i. to ℈ss. Price per lb. 28 0 0

Names, English and Country.	Botanical Names.	Remarks.
No. 79. Castoorie. Kustoorie. Castor Fiber. (?) काशतुरी کستوري		This is the name given to much adulterated musk and used only as an aphrodisiœ. Dose gr. v. to ℈i. Price per lb. 384 0 0
No. 80. Chundrus. Indian Copal. चंदरश چندرش	Vateria Indica.	Used in varnish; and its fine shavings given to check Diarrhœa. Dose ʒi. to ʒii. Price per lb. 3 0 0
No. 81. Dhunya. Coriander Seed. دهنيا	Coriandrum Sativum.	Cultivated; used as a condiment and carminative; the green plant is also eaten and called "Khotmeer." Dose ℈i to ʒi. Price per lb. 0 1 4

Names, English and Country.	Botanical Names.	Remarks.
No. 82. Dalchinee. Cinnamon. दालचीनी دالچيني	Laurus Cinnamomum.	Used as carminative and stimulant. Dose gr. v. to ℈i. Price per lb. 0 8 0
No. 83. Dal-huldi-arud. Nepal Barberry. दालहलदीआरद دارهلدي	Berberis Asiatica.	The wood is imported and used as a yellow dye; and internally as heating and carminative. Dose gr. v. to ℈i. Price per lb. 0 2 0
No. 84. Dhatoonie. داتوني	Croton Tiglium.	The bark of the root, used as a violent cathartic to produce abortion. Dose gr. v. to ℈ss. Price per lb. 2 8 0
No. 85. Dharoon-aj-ukurbie. धारुनआजआकरबी دارونج اقربي	Bambusa Nana.	Literally scorpion root, as it is very like a scorpion; the root of the cane brought from Cabul, considered tonic and aphrodisice. Dose ℈i. to ʒi. Price per lb. 24 0 0

Names, English and Country.	Botanical Names.	Remarks.
No. 86. Dhaura ka Phool. धौरा का फुल دھوریکاپھول	Grislea Tomentosa.	Indigenous; the dried flowers are considered stimulating and given to women to promote labour; used in dyeing; and the gum like tragacanth. Dose ʒss. to ʒii. Price per lb. 0 8 0
No. 87. Dhatura. धातुरा Khunuk; Khunuk ka beej. دھتورا	Datura Fastuosa and Merel.	"Kanuk," the black kind, and the seed "khunuk ka beej;" the seed is often used to poison with; smoked is excellent in asthma. Dose gr. ss. to ℈i. Price per lb. 0 3 0
No. 88. Dudiya. दुदीया دودھیا	Euphorbia Thymifolia.	Common every where; used as stimulant and laxative. Dose ℈i. to ʒi. Price per lb. 0 0 3

Names, English and Country.	Botanical Names.	Remarks.
No. 89. Dus-mooli. दसमुली دسمول		Roots of ten plants brought from Delhie and given after women's labour; used as a charm. Dose ʒii. Price per lb. 0 4 0
No. 90. Dal-shikara. दालशीरा دال چکره		Corrosive Sublimate; sometimes used in medicine; but chiefly used in "rasan," or transmutation of metals. Dose $\frac{1}{10}$ gr. Price per lb. 6 0 0
No. 91. Dal-chini-ka-tel. दालचीनी का तेल دال چيني كا تيل	Laurus Cinnamomum.	Common oil; imported both liquid and solid; used as stimulant and carminative. Dose gr. ii. to gr. v. Price per lb. 192 0 0
No. 92. Deodar. दीवदार ديودار	Pinus Deodara.	Used in incense and as febrifuge. Dose ℈i. to ʒi. Price per lb. 0 14 0

Names, English and Country.	Botanical Names.	Remarks.
No. 93. Dheriyao ka Nariyal. दरीयाव् का नारीयाल دريائي ناريل	Cocos Maldivica.	Translucent pieces of the fruit, used in fever and paralysis. Dose ℈ss. to ʒi. Price per lb. 1 8 0
No. 94. Dhookoo. धुकु Dhookoo. دوقو	Ptychotis Sylvestris.	Called also jungli jaiefull; an umbelliferus plant with a very aromatic smell, used as carminative. Dose ℈ss. to ℈ii. Price per lb. 12 0 0
No. 95. Elwa. Moosubbur. इलवा Etwa. الوة	Aloes Spicata and Erecta.	Aloes of a coarse kind; used as a purge; and externally. Dose gr. v. to ℈i. Price per lb. 0 6 0

Names, English and Country.	Botanical Names.	Remarks.
No. 96. Guj-pipur. गजपीपीख گجپیپل	Pothos Scandens. Scindapsus Officinalis.	An enormous parasitical creeper; the fruit used as carminative and tonic. Dose gr. v. to ℈i. Price per lb. 0 8 0
No. 97. Gajuba. गाजुबा گاوزبان	Anasomeles Malabarica; Ajuga Fruticosa. (?)	Catmint; purple bugle; flowers dried and capsules used as tonic and purgative. Dose ℈ss. to ʒii. Price per lb. 4 10 0
No. 98. Gokhru. गोखब گوکهرو	Tribulus Lanuginosus.	The green plant; and dried seeds and capsules highly macilaginous. Dose ʒii. to ℥i. Price per lb. 0 0 8
No. 99. Ghork-moondie. गोरखमुण्डी گورکهه مونڈي	Sphœranthus Mollis and Indica.	Indigenous; used as heating and aphrodisiac. Dose ℈ss. to ʒi. Price per lb. 0 0 8

Names, English and Country.	Botanical Names.	Remarks.
No. 100. Gundha Birosa. गनधाबीरोजः گندھا بروزہ	Bosswellia Thurifera.	Olibanum tree; imported; used in varnishes; also internally as a stimulant in ointments; and to cure gonorrhœa internally. Dose ʒss. to ʒi. Price per lb. 0 3 0
No. 101. Googul. Gum B'dellium. گوگل	Amyris Agallocha.	A gum resin; gum b'dellium, like myrrh; and used as its substitute. Plentiful at Ajmeer. Dose gr. ss. to ℈ss. Price per lb. 0 3 0
No. 102. Gari-gond. Agarikoon. आगारीकुवा غاریقون	Polyporus Igniarius.	Agaric; used as a styptic externally and internally as a bitter tonic and laxative. Dose gr. i. to gr. v. Price per lb. 26 0 0

Names, English and Country.	Botanical Names.	Remarks.
No. 103. Gao-zuban. गौजबाब گاوزبان	Cacalia Kleinia.	Dried leaves imported, used in decoction as diaphoretic and alterative. Dose ℈ss. to ʒii. in infusion. Price per lb. 4 10 0
No. 104. Gao-lochun. گاولوچن		Gall Stones; used in coloring; and also internally in jaundice. Dose gr. ss. to gr. iii. Price per lb. 96 0 0
No. 105. Gundhak. गंधाक Sulphur. گندهک		Sulphur; three kinds; ourasur gundhak, very pure, native crystals; autiya gundhak, less pure, not crystalized; nirmulasar gundhak, common roll sulphur; used to cure the itch and as a purge. Dose ʒss. to ʒii. Price per lb. 1 3 0 to 0 7 0

Names, English and Country.	Botanical Names.	Remarks.
No. 106. Gundhak ka araq. गंधाक का आरक گندهک کا عرق		Impure sulphuric acid; given internally as cooling; and used in "rasan." Dose v. to x. Price per lb. 20 0 0
No. 107. Gentiana. गइनतीआना جنتيانه	Gentiana Lutea.	Real gentian root, imported from Turkey, used as a tonic. Dose ʒi. to ʒii. in infusion. Price per lb. 2 8 0
No. 108. Gil-i-Armanie. गइलइआरमनी گل ارمني		A kind of earth, imported from Cabul; used as astringent. Dose ℈ss. to ʒss. Price per lb. 0 5 3
No. 109. Gila. गीला گلو	Mimosa Scandens.	The large seed is used in charms; and internally as aphrodisiac; and in coughs as expectorant. Dose gr. v. to ℈i. Price per lb. 0 0 8

Names, English and Country.	Botanical Names.	Remarks.
No. 110. Gool-gafiz. गुल गाफइज گل گافج	Eupatorium Cannabinum.	Hemp agrimony; used as a diluent astringent. Dose ʒss. to ʒii. in infusion. Price per lb. 6 4 0
No. 111. Goond-be-duster. Jhoonj-be-duster. गुन्दबीदस्तर Castor Fiber. جندبستر		Real Castor; imported from Cabul and used as an aphrodisiac. Dose gr. v. to ℈i. Price per lb. 630* 0 0 * One massa 1 8 0
No. 112. Gool-i-pista. गुलइपइस्ता گل پستہ	Pistacia Vera.	A kind of gall or hollow excrescence from the pistacio tree; used as astringent and resinous. Dose gr. v. to ℈i. Price per lb. 3 8 0

Names, English and Country.	Botanical Names.	Remarks.
No. 113. Gool-i-bhaboona. गुलइबाबुना Cammomile Flowers. گل‌بابونہ	Anthemis Nobilis.	Used in fevers; and given in purges. Dose gr. v. to ℈ss. Price per lb. 3 8 0
No. 114. Hub-abir. हबाबीर Juniper Berries. حب بیر	Juniperus Communis.	The dried berries brought from Nepaul; used as diuretic and to cure gonorrhœa. Dose ʒi. to ʒii. Price per lb. 0 10 0
No. 115. Hing. Assafœtida. ہینگ	Ferula Assafœtida. Narthex Assafœtida.	Largely imported, and used in food and medicine as carminative and digestive. Dose gr. ii. to ℈ss. Price per lb. 0 2 0

Names, English and Country.	Botanical Names.	Remarks.
No. 116. Hur; Hurra. হড়া Chebulic Myrobolan. هرڑ	Terminalia Chebula.	And other varieties, three in number; being all the discarded myrobolans of our old Pharmacopiœ; imported from the N. W. P., and the South. Gural Hurra, used as astringent and purgative; Jawal Hurra, used as purgative and tonic; Jangi Hurra, used as purgative and tonic; Chaipal Hurra, used only in dyeing. Dose gr. v. to ℈i. Price per lb. 0 2 0
No. 117. Hans Raj. Shair-ul-jin. হংসরাজ شعرالجين	Adian tum Capillus Veneris.	Venus's hair; grows at Patna; but, brought from Nepal; used as heating and febrifuge. Dose ℈ss. to ʒss. Price per lb. 0 5 0

Names, English and Country.	Botanical Names.	Remarks.
No. 118. Hurtal. Orpiment. हरताल Sesquisulphuret of Arsenic. هرتال		Used in painting; used internally; and in fumigations. Dose gr. $\frac{1}{16}$ Price per lb. 2 4 6
No. 119. Heera Kusees. हीरा कसीस هیراکسیس		Sulphate of iron; used in spleen, as tonic and applied externally. Dose gr. ½ to gr. ii. Price per lb. 1 10 0
No. 120. Huzrut-zahoor. Huzrut-bo. Huzrut-ool-zahood. हजरतजऊर The points of petrified Echites. حجرالوهید		Jew's stones imported from Persia. Used in charms. Dose gr. ¼ to gr. ii. Price per lb. 2 8 0

Names, English and Country.	Botanical Names.	Remarks.
No. 121. Hub-ool-kilkil. हबउलकीलकील حب کلکل	Punica Granatum.	The wild Pomegranate seed; used as cooling and astringent. Dose ʒi. to ʒii. Price per lb. 2 8 0
No. 122. Hub-ool-balsam. Carpobalsamum. हबउलबालशाम حب بلسان	Balsamodendron Gileadense.	Considered stimulant and cardiac. Dose gr. v. to ℈ss. Price per lb. 3 0 0
No. 123. Hub-ool-zelum. Hub-ool-sonden. हबउलजीलम حب الزلم	Cassia Absus.	The receptacle used as stimulant and diuretic. Dose gr. v. to ℈i. Price per lb. 3 2 0
No. 124. Hub-ool-lauztulkh. हबउललऔजतलख کڑوا بادام	Amygdalus Communis; var. Amara.	Bitter almonds, used as deobstruent. Dose ʒss. to ℥i. Price per lb. 1 4 0

Names, English and Country.	Botanical Names.	Remarks.
No. 125. Hulyoon. हलयुन هليون	Asparagus Officinalis.	The leaves, berries and roots used as demulcent and diuretic. Dose ʒii. to ℥ss. in infusion. Price per lb. 2 13 0
No. 126. Hub-ool-ghar. हबउलघार حب الغار	Laurus Nobilis.	The berries used as stimulant and tonic. Dose gr. ii. to gr. v. Price per lb. 2 2 0
No. 127. Hub-ool-khizra. हबउलखीजरा حب خزرا	Pinus Abies.	The seed of the common pine, used as tonic and diuretic. Dose ℈i. to ʒss. Price per lb. 5 0 0

Names, English and Country.	Botanical Names.	Remarks.
No. 128. Ispahgol. इस्पागोल اسپغول	Plantago Ispaghula.	The seed highly mucilagenous and very much used as a demulcent. Dose ʒii. to ℥ss. in infusion. Price per lb. 1 0 2
No. 129. Ispund. Ermul. इस्पंद اسپند	Ruta Graveolens.	Seed used in enchantments; and also considered heating; given internally as emurenagogue. Dose gr. v. to ℈i. Price per lb. 0 1 0
No. 130. Inderjau. Inderjau Shereen. इनदरजौ اندرجو	Nerium Antidysentericum. Wrightia Antidysenterica.	There are two kinds. The seeds are used, which though from different kinds of trees, differ only in being bitter and sweet. The bark of this tree is the codaga bark. The bitter seeds are given internally in dysentery and applied externally in colics; the sweet kinds are used as aphrodisiac. Dose gr. ii. to gr. viii. Price per lb. 0 12 0

Names, English and Country.	Botanical Names.	Remarks.
No. 131. Ingoor. Shengruf; Cinnabar. इंगुर انگور Persulphuret of Mercury.		Red sulphuret of mercury. Used externally and in fumigations. Dose: not given internally. Price per lb. 0 11 0
No. 132. Isquil. इसक्वील اسقل	Scilla Indica.	Indian Squill. The dried roots used as emetic and alterative. Dose gr. ½ to ℈i. Price per lb. 0 4 0
No. 133. Ish-khess. इसखेस اسخس	Daphne Viridiflora.	The seed and bark of the roots used as stimulant and sudorific, and act like mezereon. Dose gr. ½ to gr. iii. Price per lb. 0 13 0

Names, English and Country.	Botanical Names.	Remarks.
No. 134. Jal-lakri. जललकरी Billilotan. جل‌لکري	Valeriana Paludosa.	Wild Valerian. The whole plant dried used in scents; and as refrigerant. Dose ʒss. to ʒi. Price per lb. 0 1 0
No. 135. Jamalgoota. जमालगोटा جمالگوٹه	Croton Tiglium.	And several other species; the seeds are used, made into pills with ginger and kutkaranja seeds; and are a violent purge. Dose gr. $\frac{1}{6}$ to gr. iii. Price per lb. 0 8 0
No. 136. Jowa Khar. जोवाखार جواکهار	Hordeum Hexastychon.	Ashes of the barley leaves; used as cooling in sherbets. Dose ʒii. to ℥ss. Price per lb. 0 3 0
No. 137. Jadwar. Nirbishee. जादवार جدوار	Curcuma Zedoaria.	Considered heating; used also in scents: one kind imported kept in oil and used only externally. Dose gr. ii. to gr. v. Price per lb. 2 8 0

Names, English and Country.	Botanical Names.	Remarks.
No. 138. Joufa; Jufiah. जुफा جوفيا	Croton Joufia.	The dried plant considered heating and used in coughs. Dose gr. ½ to gr. v. Price per lb. 0 10 0
No. 139. Jungal. जंगाल Sub-acetate of Copper. زنگار		Sub-acetate of Copper, used externally in ointments. Dose: not given internally. Price per lb. 1 0 0
No. 140. Jahur-moora-kutai. जाहर मुरा षटै Very pure Steatite. زهرمهرهٔ خطائي		A kind of steatite, given as an anti-nauseant in cholera. Dose ℈ii. to ʒiss. Price per lb. 1 4 0
No. 141. Jatamansie. जातामानसी جٹاماسي	Valeriana Jatamansie.	A kind of spikenard imported from Nepal and used in scents: and which differs both from the Balchur and Kurphus. Used as refrigerant. Dose gr. v. to ℈i. Price per lb. 1 4 0

Names, English and Country.	Botanical Names.	Remarks.
No. 142. Jawe-sheer. जावीशीर جواشیر	Opoponax Chironium.	Gum Opoponax. Used as a stimulant internally and externally. Dose gr. ii. to ℈ss. Price per lb. 5 0 0
No. 143. Jalapa. जलापा جلاپه	Convolvulus Xalapa.	Real Jaláp Root; sold in irregular dried pieces in the Bazars; imported; and very impure. Dose gr. iii. to ℈ii. Price per lb. 15 0 0
No. 144. Kuth. कथ کتهه	Acacia Catechu.	Japan Earth; universally used as astringent and tonic. Dose ʒ ss. to ℈ii. Price per lb. 0 4 0
No. 145. Kaephul. कैफल کایپهل	Myrica Sapida.	The bark imported from the Hills, and used as an excellent external stimulant. Dose: not given internally. Price per lb. 0 3 0

Names, English and Country.	Botanical Names.	Remarks.
No. 146. Koot. Differs wholly from the real Koot or Putchuk. कुट كوٹ	Costus Arabicus.	Root of the plant found near water, used in messalas, inodorous and tasteless. Dose ℈ii. to ʒii. Price per lb. 0 2 0
No. 147. Kala-jeera. Kooksheem. कालाजीरा Blue Flea Bane. كالي زيري	Vernonia Cinerea. Conyza Cinerea. Serratula Cinerea.	The seed strongly scented and used as an alexipharmic and in messalas of horses, also as authelmintic. Dose gr. v. to ℈ii. Price per lb. 0 1 0
No. 148. Kesur. Zaffran. Saffron. केशर زعفران	Crocus Sativus.	Imported and used as an aromatic and stimulant. Dose ℈ss. to ℈ii. Price per lb. 25 0 0
No. 149. Kakra Singh. काकरशिंघ ككڑا سنگهي	Rhus Acuminata.	The hollow galls of the tree used as very astringent. Dose gr. iii. to ℈ss. Price per lb. 0 10 0

Names, English and Country.	Botanical Names.	Remarks.
No. 150. Kiwanch. कोवांच کیوانچهه	Mucuna Pruritus. Dolichos Pruriens.	The seeds only are used as aphrodisiac. Dose gr. ii. to gr. v. Price per lb. 0 2 0
No. 151. Kantala. कानटाला Cantula. کنٹهاله	Fourcroyia Cantula.	The infusion of the dried leaves is given to promote diaphoresis in coughs and fevers. Dose gr. viii. to ℈i. in infusion. Price per lb. 0 2 0
No. 152. Kulinjan. Galangale. कुलइनजन کولنجن	Alpinia Galanga.	The root very fragrant, aromatic and bitter; used to promote digestion and in fevers. Dose gr. iii. to ℈ss. Price per lb. 0 10 0
No. 153. Katila ka gond. कतीला का गोंद کتیلا کا گوند	Sterculia Urens.	An enormous tree; also obtained from the Grislea Tomentosa. Both gums are exactly like Tragacanth. Demulcent. Dose ℈i. to ʒii. Price per lb. 0 2 0

Names, English and Country.	Botanical Names.	Remarks.
No. 154. Khar-suji. खार सुजी Suji Khar. كهارسجي	Salsola Indica.	Impure Soda imported from Sinde; full of charcoal, used to make soap, also glass; and applied externally to discuss tumours. Dose: not given internally. Price per lb. 0 1 0
No. 155. Kuchla. कुचला كوچله	Strychnos Nux Vomica.	The seed is sold in great abundance, and is chiefly used as an aphrodisiac. Dose gr. $\frac{1}{16}$ to ℨss. Price per lb. 0 12 0
No. 156. Khasnie ka jur. कासनी का जड़ كاسني كا جڑ	Cichorium Endivium.	Indian Succory Root; used as demulcent. Dose ℨii. to ℥i. in infusion. Price per lb. 0 3 4
No. 157. Kureel. करील كريل	Capparis Aphylla. Capparis Acuminata.	Indian Leafless Caper Tree. The buds are used in pickles; and eaten dried to stimulate digestion. Dose ℈i. to ℨss. Price per lb. 0 1 2

Names, English and Country.	Botanical Names.	Remarks.
No. 158. Kulfi. कुलफी قلفه	Portulaca Oleracea.	Seed used as cooling and astringent in drinks. Dose ʒii. to ℥ss. in infusion. Price per lb. 0 1 6
No. 159. Kupila. कपीला کپیله	Rottlera Tinctoria.	The dust from the Capsule of the fruit is used to dye silk yellow; considered as of a warm nature, and given internally as anthelmintic. Dose gr. ii. to gr. v. Price per lb. 0 3 0
No. 160. Kaphoor Kuchri. काफुर कचरी کپورکچري	Hedychium Spicatum.	Lesser Galangale. The root fragrant, warm and aromatic; and so used. Dose gr. v. to ℈ii. Price per lb. 0 2 0
No. 161. Kesru. Hursingar. केसर هرسنگهار	Nyctanthes arbor Tristis.	The yellow tubes of the corolœ are used in dyeing; and also given internally in dysmenorrhœa. Dose gr. v. to ℈i. Price per lb. 0 6 0

Names, English and Country.	Botanical Names.	Remarks.
No. 162. Kath Karanja. काथ करानजः كتكرنجا	Cœsalpinia Bonducella.	The Nicker Tree. The seed is the Bonduc Nut; and used as a febrifuge and tonic. Dose gr. ii. to ℈ss. Price per lb. 0 0 8
No. 163. Khatmi. कायमी خطمي	Malva Sylvestris.	Marsh mallow—the seed used as demulcent. Dose ʒii. to ℥ss. in infusion. Price per lb. 0 5 0
No. 164. Khoombaji. Chota-gool Khairu. खुभाजी خبازي	Althœa Alhugas.	Common dwarf mallow, used in the same way. Dose ʒii. to ℥ss. in infusion. Price per lb. 0 1 6
No. 165. Khoob Kalam. खुब कालाम Debun Sha. Sweet Basil Seed. خوبكلان	Ocimum Basilicum.	Used as an aphrodisiac. Dose ʒss. to ℥iii. Price per lb. 0 3 4

Names, English and Country.	Botanical Names.	Remarks.
No. 166. Kathir Ranga. काथीर كتهر رانگا		Tin, used in the state of oxide as a tonic and aphrodisiac. Dose gr. ⅛ to gr. ii. Price per lb. 0 8 0
No. 167. Kalmi Sora. कालमी शोरा قلمي شوره		Nitrate of Potash. Given internally as cooling in gonorrhœas and fevers. Dose gr. ii. to gr. v. Price per lb. 0 1 4
No. 168. Kora-chal. कोराचाल Codaga Bark. خوراچهال	Wrightia Antidysenterica.	The bark of the tree from the N. W. P., very bitter; used as tonic and sudorific. Dose gr. iii. to gr. viii. Price per lb. 0 1 4
No. 169. Kak-nuj. काकनज كاكنج	Physalis Flexuosa.	The seed of the flexible winter cherry used as diuretic and hypnotic. Dose gr. v. to ʒii. in infusion. Price per lb. 2 2 8½

Names, English and Country.	Botanical Names.	Remarks.
No. 170. Khair Sar. खैर सार خیرسار	Acacia Catechu.	Grains of astringent matter from the heart of the wood of the tree. Dose gr. v. to ℈ii. Price per lb. 0 5 0
No. 171. Kala Nimuk. काला नमक کالانمک		Black salt, much used and eaten to promote digestion. Dose gr. v. to gr. xv. Price per lb. 0 2 0
No. 172. Kaladana. कालादाना کالادانہ	Ipomœa Cœrulœa. Pharbitis Cœrulœa.	The black seed is used half roasted as a purge. Dose ℈ss. to ʒiss. Price per lb. 0 2 0
No. 173. Kukrot. काकरोट Ukroot. ککروٹ	Aleurites Triloba.	A hard stony seed; the almond eaten as stimulant and sudorific. Dose ʒii. to ℥i. Price per lb. 0 4 0

Names, English and Country.	Botanical Names.	Remarks.
No. 174. Kaphoor. Camphor. कापुर کافور	Laurus Camphora.	Much used as a stimulant both internally and externally. Dose gr. ¼ to gr. viii. Price per lb. 1 3 0
No. 175. Kala-megh. Maha Tita. Creat ka jur. कालमेघ کالامیگ	Andrographis Paniculata.	The root used as a stomachic bitter; and in the "drogue amere." Dose ʒss. to ʒi. in infusion. Price per lb. 3 8 0
No. 176. Koosht-tulkh. Putchuk Root. The real Koot. कुश्त तलख کوشت تلخ	Aucklandia Costus.	The bitter is called koosht-tulk; and the sweet koosht-shereen; the roots have a fragrant smell and are used in scents; and as refrigerant. Dose ℈i. to ʒii. Price per lb. 0 5 0

Names, English and Country.	Botanical Names.	Remarks.
No. 177. Kashim. काशीम كاشم	Ferula Assafœtida. Narthex Assafœtida.	Assafœtida. Seed and leaves of the plant considered sudorific and carminative. Dose ℈ss. to ʒii. Price per lb. 3 2 0
No. 178. Kamraj. कामराज كامراج		The root is used like that of Bhidaira as restorative and aphrodisiac. Dose gr. ii. to ℈ii. Price per lb. 0 4 0
No. 179. Khorasanie Kootki. खोराशानी कुटकी خراساني كٹكي	Helleborus Niger and Albus.	The roots of Black and White Hellebores; used as drastic cathartics to cause abortion. Dose gr. ii. to ℈i. Price per lb. 1 0 0
No. 180. Kahroba Poorbie. Amber. काहरोबा كهربة		Used as an aphrodisiac. Dose gr. ii. to ℈ss. Price per lb. 8 0 0

Names, English and Country.	Botanical Names.	Remarks.
No. 181. Kahroba Mugurwi. काहरोबा मगरबी كهربه مغربي		Another kind of amber brought from the West, used as aphrodisiac. Dose gr. ii. to ℈ss. Price per lb. 8 0 0
No. 182. Koondur Roomie. Roomie Mastungi. कुंदर रुमी رومي مستكي	Pistacia Lentiscus.	Mastich used as an astringent internally. Dose gr. ii. to gr. xv. Price per lb. 3 2 0
No. 183. Kuntraoon. कांदाउन كنتريون	Eragrostis Purpurascens.	The small seeds, and stalks are very wooly, and used as a diluent. Dose ʒii. to ℥ss. in infusion. Price per lb. 2 8 0
No. 184. Kupuriya. कपरीया كهپريا		Semivitrified clay mixed with oxides of several metals; probably the remains of cupels; considered poisonous; used as aphrodisiac. Dose gr. $\frac{1}{16}$ to gr. $\frac{1}{2}$. Price per lb. 0 8 0

Names, English and Country.	Botanical Names.	Remarks.
No. 185. Kadishen. कादीशीन کادیشین	Cluytia Collina.	The Pericarp is poisonous; and is used as aphrodisiac. Dose gr. $\frac{1}{4}$ to gr. i. Price per lb. 2 4 0
No. 186. Kaka-todali. काकातोदाली کاکاتودلي	Toddalia Aculeata.	The bark is used as astringent and tonic; the seed is heating. Dose gr. v. to gr. xv. Price per lb. 1 10 0
No. 187. Kak mari ka beej. काक मारी का बीज کاکماري کا بیج	Anamirta paniculata. Cocculus Indicus.	The seeds are used as excitants and aphrodisiac; and to poison with. Dose gr. $\frac{1}{8}$ to gr. i. Price per lb. 3 8 0
No. 188. Kamaranga. Harpharewrie. कामारंगा کامارنگا	Averrhœa Carambola.	The acid dried fruit given in fevers. Dose ʒi. to ℥i. Price per lb. 0 0 6

Names, English and Country.	Botanical Names.	Remarks.
No. 189. Kamela. कामीला کمیله	Daphne Mezereon.	The seed imported from Cabul; and used as an irritant. Dose gr. ¼ to gr. iii. Price per lb. 5 0 0
No. 190. Kunghai. काँघै کنگهي	Sida graveolens.	The root used as bitter and diaphoretic. Dose ʒss. to ʒii. in infusion. Price per lb. 0 2 0
No. 191. Kundel. Sagapenum. कनडेल کندیل	Ferula Sagapenum.	Used externally; also given as a stimulant. Dose gr. ¼ to ℈ss. Price per lb. 5 0 0
No. 192. Khul-ka-jur. खुल का जड़ خول کا جر	Œrua Lanata Achyranthes Lanata.	Root used as demulcent. Dose ʒii. to ℥i. in infusion. Price per lb. 0 2 0

Names, English and Country.	Botanical Names.	Remarks.
No. 193. Kurabik. Kanel. कनेल Khurrabhee. كربق	Nerium Odorum.	Bark of the root poisonous; externally discutient. Dose: not used internally medicinally. Price per lb. 0 1 0
No. 194. Kurufs. करफश كرفس	Apium Graveolens.	Celery; the seed used as carminative. Dose ℈ss. to ʒss. Price per lb. 2 8 0
No. 195. Kushoos. Kushoos Roomie. कसुष كشوش رومي	Cuscutta Europœa.	Dodder worm-wood; used as diaphoretic. Dose gr. ¼ to gr. iss. Price per lb. 0 10 0
No. 196. Kahoo. Khuss ka beej Lettuce seed. काहू کاهو	Lactuca Sativa.	The seed used as demulcent. Dose ʒii. to ℥ss. in infusion. Price per lb. 0 2 0

Names, English and Country.	Botanical Names.	Remarks.
No. 197. Kermez. कोरमीज् كرمس	Coccus Baphica.	The dried insects are used in dyeing; and given in dysmenorrhœa. Dose gr. ss. to gr. viii. Price per lb. 5 0 0
No. 198. Kootki. कूटकी كٹكي	Picrorrhiza Kurrooa.	Roots used as a tonic in purges. Dose gr. ¼ to gr. ii. Price per lb. 0 2 0
No. 199. Keysoo. केसु كيسو	Anthoxan thum Nepalense.	An odoriferous grass used in scents as refrigerant. Dose ℈i. to ʒss. Price per lb. 0 5 0
No. 200. Kuchnar. काचनार كچنار	Bauhinia Variegata.	The bark is used as tonic in fevers. Dose gr. v. to ℈i. Price per lb. 0 1 0

Names, English and Country.	Botanical Names.	Remarks.
No. 201. Lodh. लोध لودہ	Symplocos Racemosa.	The bark is used in dyeing, and also given to promote the flow of the menses. Dose ℈ii. to ʒiss. Price per lb. 0 0 8
No. 202. Lila Tootiya. लीला तुतीया ليلاتوتيا		Sulphate of Copper, used as an escharotic only. Dose: not given medicinally by the native medical men. Price per lb. 0 5 3
No. 203. Lil-ka-phool. लील का फुल ليل کا پھول	Indigofera Anil.	The flowers and leaves are given in disease of the liver and bowels. Dose ʒii. to ℥i. in infusion. Price per lb. 0 1 0
No. 204. Loban. लोबान لوبان	Styrax Benzoin.	Gum Benjamin, used in incense; and applied externally; also used as an aphrodisiac. Dose gr. v. to ℈i. Price per lb. 3 0 0

Names, English and Country.	Botanical Names.	Remarks.
No. 205. Laj burud. Lapis Lazuli. लाजबरद لاجورد		Used as an astringent and refrigerant; also in painting. Dose gr. v. to ℈i. Price per lb. 10 0 0
No. 206. Long-ka-tel. लोंग का तेल لونگ کا تیل	Engenia Caryophyllata.	Oil of Cloves; used as a stimulant. Dose i. to v. Price per lb. 60 0 0
No. 207. Laj-aloo. लाज आलु لاجالو	Mimosa Natans.	Water sensitive plant, used as refrigerant and astringent. Dose ℈ii. to ʒii. Price per lb. 0 1 0
No. 208. Lahorie Hoormul. लहोरी हरमल لاهوري هرمل	Ruta Albiflora Peganum Harmala.	White Rue. The whole plant used as a stimulant. Dose gr. v. to ʒss. Price per lb. 0 3 6

Names, English and Country.	Botanical Names.	Remarks.
No. 209. Lufah. लुफा لوفه	Mandragora Officinalis.	The fruit of the mandrake; used as narcotic. Dose gr. $\frac{1}{8}$ to gr. $\frac{1}{2}$. Price per lb. 0 10 0
No. 210. Lasora. लाश्चोरा لسوره	Cordia Myxa.	The dried fruit used as demulcent and restorative. Dose ℥ss. to ℥i. Price per lb. 0 2 0
No. 211. Lil. Indigo. लील ليل	Indigofera Tinctoria. Indigofera Officinalis.	Used to bad ulcers; especially in horses. Dose: not given internally. Price per lb. 3 2 0
No. 212. Lal. Small Rubies. लाल لعل		Used medicinally, as aphrodisiac. Dose gr. $\frac{1}{2}$ to gr. v. Price per lb. 30 0 0

Names, English and Country.	Botanical Names	Remarks.
No. 213. Lis-an ool As-ufeer. Inderjau Tulkh. लीसान उल असाफीर لسان الاسافیر	Holarrhena Pubescen; and Antidysenterica.	The bitter pods of this tree used in dysenteries and fevers; as tonic and sudorific; and applied externally in colics. Imported kind. Dose gr. ii. to gr. v. Price per lb. 0 8 0
No. 214. Loheck. लोहीक لوحق	Ophiorrhiza Mungos.	The root sold as a charm for snake bites. Dose: not given internally. Price per lb. 20 0 0
No. 215. Ladan. Labdanum. लादान لادن	Cistus Creticus.	Used externally; and as an aphrodisiac. Dose gr. ii. to ℈ss. Price per lb. 120 0 0
No. 216. Lunka-sij. लंकासीज لنکاسیج	Euphorbia Tirucalli.	The acrid juice is applied externally to ulcers. Dose: not given internally. Price per lb. 0 1 0

Names, English and Country.	Botanical Names.	Remarks.
No. 217. Loha-ka-Lochun. लोहा का लोचन لوہا کا لوچن		Iron filings used as a tonic. Dose gr. ¼ to gr. ii. Price per lb. 0 2 0
No. 218. Lublab. लबलाब لبلاب	Hedera Helix.	Ivy leaves; used to stimulate sores; and the berries to purge. Dose gr. ii. to gr. v. Price per lb. 0 10 0
No. 219. Lisan-ool-kulb. लइसान उल कलब لسان الکلب	Cynoglossum Officinale.	Dog's Tongue; the seed is used as mucilaginous and astringent. Dose ℈ii. to ʒii. in infusion. Price per lb. 5 0 0
No. 220. Lisan-ool-heml. लइसान उल हमल لسان الحمل	Plantago Afra. Arnoglossum.	Weruck Bartung-Plantago. The seed used as demulcent and refrigerant. Dose ʒi. to ℥ss. in infusion. Price per lb. 5 0 0

Names, English and Country.	Botanical Names.	Remarks.
No. 221. Maida-lakri. मैदालाकरी ميده‌لكري	Tetranthera Roxburghii.	The bark and wood of this large tree brought from the N. W. P., applied to wounds; and used as aphrodisiac. Dose ℈ii. to ʒiss. Price per lb. 0 2 0
No. 222. Muslie-sufaid. मुसली सफेद مصلي‌سفيد	Bombax Heptaphyllum. Salmalia Malabarica.	The root used as stimulating in purges and messalas; but is chiefly mucilaginous. Dose ʒi. to ʒii. in infusion. Price per lb. 0 2 0
No. 223. Muslie siyah. मुसली सीया مصلي‌سياه	This root has activity and belongs to a different genus doubtless.	The root is used as aphrodisiac; also emetic. Dose ℈ss. to ℈ii. Price per lb. 0 2 0
No. 224. Muraiti-ka-jur. मरहैटी का जड़ ميريٹي کا جڑ	Glycyrrhiza Glabra.	The extract called rub-us-soos is used as a demulcent. Dose gr. v. to ʒss. Price per lb. 0 5 4

Names, English and Country.	Botanical Names.	Remarks.
No. 225. Munsa-sij. मनशाशीज منساسيج	Euphorbia Ligularia.	The root mixed with stimulants is given in snake bites. Dose gr. ii. to gr. v. Price per lb. 0 1 0
No. 226. Makoe. मकोइ مكوئي	Smilax Prolifera.	A species of sarsaparilla, very common in the Dekkhan; the small black berries are eaten; the root is used in decoction. Dose ℥ss. to ℥ii. in decoction. Price per lb. 0 8 0
No. 227. Mako. Tulidun; Ghurki. माको مكو	Solanum Nigrum and Rubrum.	The dried berries of both are eaten; the leaves are given in colics; the leaves and roots are used in decoction, as fomentations. Dose ʒii. to ℥ss. Price per lb. 0 2 0

Names, English and Country.	Botanical Names.	Remarks.
No. 228. Mooltanie mittie. ملتاني متّي		A kind of light yellow ochre; eaten in dyspepsia in small quanties. Dose gr. v. to ℈ss. Price per lb. 0 0 6
No. 229. Methi. मेथी Hœnugreeb. متهي	Trigonella Fœnum Græcum.	The seed is very much used in medicine as stimulant and carminative. Dose ℈ss. to ʒi. Price per lb. 0 0 8
No. 230. Malkhagni. मालखागनी مالكگني	Celastrus Paniculatus.	The seeds are considered sudorific. An empyreumatic oil is distilled and given internally as stimulant. Dose gr. iss. to gr. iii. Price per lb. 0 2 0
No. 231. Maror-phulli. मारोरफली مرورپهلي	Helicteres Isora.	The twisted pods are used as a charm in colic. Dose ℈ss. to ʒi. Price per lb. 0 2 0

Names, English and Country.	Botanical Names.	Remarks.
No. 232. Munjisth. Chol Munjeet. मनजीष्ठ منجیتهه	Rubia Munjeeta.	Indian madder; used in dyeing, the whole plant; and given in dysmenorrhœa. Dose ℈i. to ʒiss. Price per lb. 0 3 0
No. 233. Mainphull. मैनफल مین پهل	Vanguiera Spinosa.	The dried fruit is intoxicating, and emetic. Dose gr. ½ to ℈i. Price per lb. 0 8 0
No. 234. Moordar Sung. मुरदार शंग مُردارسنگ		Semivitrified oxide of Lead, much used to all sores; also taken as a tonic. Dose gr. ⅛ to gr. ¼ Price per lb. 0 3 0
No. 235. Mainsill. मैनशइल منسل		An orange and yellow sulphuret of arsenic composed of orpiment and realgar, given in itch and other complaints. Dose gr. $\frac{1}{16}$ to gr. $\frac{1}{10}$ Price per lb. 5 0 0

Names, English and Country.	Botanical Names.	Remarks.
No. 236. Moongas ka jur. मुंगास का जड़ مونگاس کا جڑ	Solanum Spirale.	A middle sized root from the N. W. P. and given as narcotic and diuretic. Dose gr. ¼ to gr. viii. Price per lb. 0 8 0
No. 237. Moongay ka jur. मुंगे का जड़ Gigantic Mustard Tree. مونگی کا جڑ	Hyperanthera Moringa.	The root is used in debility and as an aphrodisiac; and is exactly like horse radish; is diuretic. Dose ℈i. to ʒiii. Price per lb. 0 1 0
No. 238. Muti-buka. मोतीबुका موتي بکا		Small pearls used as aphrodisiac. Dose gr. i. to ℈ss. Price per lb. 600 0 0
No. 239. Maju-phull. माजुफाल ماجوپھل	Quercus Infectoria.	Gall Nuts much used externally and in dyeing: also given as astringent. Dose gr. i. to ℈i. Price per lb. 1 2 0

Names, English and Country.	Botanical Names.	Remarks.
No. 240. Mor-punkhee. मोरपंखी مورپنکهي	Asplenium Radiatum.	Peacock's Tail. A plant (a fern) from the N. W. P., used as anthelmintic. Dose gr. iss. to ℈ss. Price per lb. 1 4 0
No. 241. Maida ka choor. मैदा का चुर ميدهکچور	Curcuma Rubescens.	The root brought from the N. W. P., has a sweet smell; and is considered refrigerant. Dose ℈ss. to ʒss. Price per lb. 0 2 0
No. 242. Mai-shutr-arabi. मैशटरआराबी ماهي‌ستر‌عربي		The blood of a young camel coagulated and dried; used in impotency. Dose gr. viii. to ʒss. Price per lb. 20 0 0
No. 243. Mahee rubiya. माही रबीया ماهي روبيا		A dried fish brought from the N. W. P., used in impotency. The flying fish (?) often dried shrimps. Dose ℥ss. to ℥i. Price per lb. 15 0 0

Names, English and Country.	Botanical Names.	Remarks.
No. 244. Mooli-khar. मुळीखार مولي کهار	Raphanus Sativus.	Radish ashes; used in indigestion. Dose ℈ii. to ʒii. Price per lb. 1 8 0
No. 245. Mochrus. मोचीरस موچرس	Salmalia Malabarica. Bombax Heptaphyllum.	The gum of the Semul Tree, given to children as a laxative. Dose gr. v. to ℈ii. Price per lb. 0 3 0
No. 246. Mushuk. Musk. मुश्क مسک اصل Moschus Moschiferus.		Very rarely to be had pure, used in impotency, also in scents. Dose gr. viii. to ℈i. Price per lb. 420 0 0
No. 247. Machootie. माचुटी مهاچهوتي	Polygonum Aviculare.	The fruit used as emetic and cathartic. Dose gr. iii. to ℈i. Price per lb. 0 1 0

Names, English and Country.	Botanical Names.	Remarks.
No. 248. Mahaburee Butch Nar-ka-choor. माहाबरी बच مهبري بچهه	Zingiber Zerumbet.	Used as a stimulant and tonic. Dose gr. iii. to ʒss. Price per lb. 1 8 0
No. 249. Makal. माकाल ماكل	Trichosanthes Palmata.	Applied as a discutient externally. Dose: not given internally. Price per lb. 0 1 0
No. 250. Murroo. मरु مرو	Origanum Majorana.	The dried plant used in scents and as a stimulant. Dose gr. v. to ℈ii. Price per lb. 0 14 0
No. 251. Maeen-burrie. माइनबड़ी ماين بڑي	Tamarix Gallica.	The astringent fruit; used in decoction. Dose ℈ii. to ʒii. Price per lb. 0 3 0

Names, English and Country.	Botanical Names.	Remarks.
No. 252. Maeen-chotie. माइनचोटी ماين چهوٹي	Tamarix Furas.	A smaller kind of similar fruit used in the same way. Dose ℈ii. to ʒii. Price per lb. 0 3 0
No. 253. Muhmooda. मह्मुदा Sunk mooniya. محموده	Convolvulus Scammonia.	Scammony of two kinds; used in purges. Dose gr. iss. to gr. viii. Price per lb. 5 0 0
No. 254. Maha-bhurree-mugurvi. महाभरीमगरबी مهبري مغربي	Zingiber Piperitum.	The root fragrant and very hot and aromatic; used as a stimulant. Dose gr. iii. to ℈i. Price per lb. 0 4 0
No. 255. Mogra Chaul. Chaul Mogra. चावल मोगरी موگرا چاول	Gynocardia Odorata. Chaulmogra Odorata.	The seeds used rubbed up to apply to the itch, given internally, are emetic and poisonous. Dose gr. $\frac{1}{16}$ to gr. $\frac{1}{4}$ Price per lb. 0 2 0

Names, English and Country.	Botanical Names.	Remarks.
No. 256. Mameera. मामीरा ماميران	Daphnee Mezereon.	This root is like mezereon and used in the same way. Dose ℈ss. to ℈ii. in decoction. Price per lb. 38 0 0
No. 257. Merjan-goosh. मरजानगुश مرزان گوش	Hieracium Pilosella.	The leaves and stalks of the plant used as tonic and astringent. Dose ℈i. to ʒi. Price per lb. 2 8 0
No. 258. Munjhoo rookha. Kukronda. मनजु रुखा منجھوروکھه	Pluchea Indica.	The root and leaves are used in fevers and as an astringent. Dose ℈i. to ʒii. in infusion. Price per lb. 0 10 0
No. 259. Mowa-ka-bukul. मोवा का बकल مهوه کا بکل	Bassia Latifolia.	The bark used in decoction as astringent and tonic. Dose ℈ii. to ʒii. Price per lb. 0 2 0

Names, English and Country.	Botanical Names.	Remarks.
No. 260. Missee. मइशी مسي		White and black missee; the white is pounded double refracting spar: the black is sulphate of iron and astringent. Dose: applied to the gums. Price per lb. 1 4 0
No. 261. Nasadar. नौशादर نوسادر		Muriate of Ammonia, used externally. Dose: not given internally. Price per lb. 0 4 0
No. 262. Nag keshur. नागकेशर ناگ کیسر	Mesua Ferrea.	The dried Pistils are used like saffron in scents and messallas; and the berries in fevers. Dose gr. vi. to ℈i. Price per lb. 0 8 0
No. 263. Nak-chikni. नाकचीकनी ناکچهکني	Hoya Viridiflora.	Used in colds and eye disease to cause sneezing. Dose gr. i. to ℈ss. Price per lb. 0 8 0

Names, English and Country.	Botanical Names.	Remarks.
No. 264. Nugur Motha. नगर मोथा ناگرموتهه	Cyperus Juncifolius.	The roots used in scents, also as diuretic and sudorific. Dose ℈i. to ʒii. Price per lb. 0 1 0
No. 265. Nirmali ka beej. नीरमली का बीज نرملي کا بيج	Strychnos Potatorum.	The seeds used to clear water; and applied externally. Dose: not given internally. Price per lb. 0 12 0
No. 266. Neem-gilo. Gulancha. नीमगीलो نیم گلو	Menispermum Cordifolium. Cocculus Cordifolius.	The stem, leaves, root, and extract are used. It is intensely bitter and taken in fevers and cutaneous diseases. Dose gr. $\frac{1}{4}$ to gr. viii. Price per lb. 0 12 0
No. 267. Nafirman. नाफाइरमान نافرمان	Dilphinium Ajacis.	Seed very acrid, emetic and cathartic. Dose gr. $\frac{1}{8}$ to gr. iii. Price per lb. 1 8 0

Names, English and Country.	Botanical Names.	Remarks.
No. 268. Nagdowna. नागदोवन ناگدونا	Artemisia Indica.	Leaves used in decoction as tonics. Dose ʒss. to ℥ss. Price per lb. 0 3 0
No. 269. Nasbo. नाशबो ناسبو	Ocimum Pilosum.	The dried leaves are used as sternutatory. Dose: not given internally. Price per lb. 0 2 0
No. 270. Naspal. नाशपाल ناسپال	Punica Granatum.	The capsule used as astringent in medicine and in dyeing. Dose gr. iii. to ℈ii. Price per lb. 0 2 0
No. 271. Neela-ghiria. Kalizar-ka-jur. Uparajita. नीलाघोड़ीया نیلاگریا	Clitorea Ternatea.	The root used as emetic. Dose ℈i. to ʒii. in decoction. Price per lb. 0 3 0

Names, English and Country.	Botanical Names.	Remarks.
No. 272. Neemooka. नीमुका نیموکا	Cissampelos Hexandra.	The root tonic, diuretic, and sudorific; scarce at Patna and little used. Dose ʒi. to ℥ss. in decoction. Price per lb. 7 7 0
No. 273. Nishinda. Nirgoondi. नीश्नीदा نیشند	Vitex Negundo.	The berries heating; the leaves aromatic; and used in decoction in fevers. Dose ℈ii. to ʒii. in infusion. Price per lb. 0 2 0
No. 274. Neem-ka-bukul. नीम का बकल نیم کا بکل	Melia Azederachta.	The bark intensely bitter and used in fevers. Dose ℈ii. to ℥ss. in infusion. Price per lb. 0 1 0
No. 275. Nar-kewa. Khus-khass Sabeedie. नारकेवा نارکیوه	Papaver Album.	The capsules are used as sedatives; imported. Dose ℈. to ʒi. in infusion. Price per lb. 2 8 0

Names, English and Country.	Botanical Names.	Remarks.
No. 276. Narfaris. नारफारइस نارفارس	Cochlospermum Gossypinum.	Dried leaves and flowers used as stimulants. Dose ℈i. to ʒii. in infusion. Price per lb. 5 0 0
No. 277. Nardeen. Nard. नारदीन ناردین	Valeriana Celtica.	A scented root from Turkey;—very like but not the same as Balchur and Jatamansic. Used in the same way ; much dearer. Dose gr. v. to ℈i. Price per lb. 5 0 0
No. 278. Neelufar. नीलुफार نیلوفر	Nymphœa Cyanea.	The dried flowers used in decoction ; as sudorific. Dose ℈ss. to ℈ii. Price per lb. 0 10 0
No. 279. Nukachoonie. नकाचुनी ناکچني	Stemodia Viscosa.	The dried plant slightly fragrant and mucilagenous; used as demulcent. Dose ℈ii. to ℥ss. in infusion. Price per lb. 2 10 0

Names, English and Country.	Botanical Names.	Remarks.
No. 280. Nuful. नफ़ल نفل	Cenchrus Echinatus.	This dried grass used as diuretic and diluent. Dose ℈ii. to ℥ss. in infusion. Price per lb. 0 8 0
No. 281. Oosara rewund. उसारा रेवन्द عصارہ ریوند	Stalagmites Gambogioides.	Gamboge, used as a drastic purgative, also applied externally. Dose gr. $\frac{1}{10}$ to gr. v. Price per lb. 3 12 0
No. 282. Ootingum ka beej. उटंगन का बीज اوتنگن کا بیج	Urtica Crenulata.	The seed like coriander, is used in the same way. This is the seed of one of the large acrid nettles very common in Nepaul. Dose ℈ss. to ℥ss. Price per lb. 0 8 0
No. 283. Oosta khudoos. उसटा खदुस اسطخدوس	Lavendula Stæchas.	The dried plant used in scents and messalas and as refrigerant. Dose ℈ii. to ℥ss. in infusion. Price per lb. 3 12 0

Names, English and Country.	Botanical Names.	Remarks.
No. 284. Oodrooz. Oodrus. उदरूज عودروج		A yellowish white gum; used to apply to the forehead in head aches. Dose: not given internally. Price per lb. 5 0 0
No. 285. Oodsaleeb. उदसालीब عودثالب	Orchis Longicornu.	The roots brought from Persia, used as astringent and diaphoretic. Dose gr. v. to ℈i. Price per lb. 1 4 0
No. 286. Oosbo Mugurwie. उश्बो मगरवी عشبة مغربي	Smilax Sarsa (?)	Thé root exactly resembles sarsaparilla and is used the same way; said also to be the long pendulous dried roots of the Banyan tree. Dose ʒii. to ℈ii. in decoction. Price per lb. 3 8 0
No. 287. Ooshuk. Ushuk. उश्शक عُشق	Dorema Ammoniacum.	Gum Ammonia; used in coughs; and applied externally. Dose gr. $\frac{1}{2}$ to gr. vi. Price per lb. 2 12 0

Names, English and Country.	Botanical Names.	Remarks.
No. 288. Ooda Chereytta. उदा चीरेटा اُوداچريتا	Exacum Tetragonum.	The root used as bitter and tonic. Dose gr. v. to ʒss. Price per lb. 0 4 0
No. 289. Ood-ool-humul. उदउलहूमल عودالحمل	Lycopodium Hookeri.	Used as stimulant and narcotic. Dose gr. ¼ to gr. iii. Price per lb. 7 9 0
No. 290. Ood-bulsan. उदबालश्रान عودبلسان	Balsamodendron Gileadense.	The wood scented; and used as a stimulant. Dose ℈ss. to ʒss. Price per lb. 2 8 0
No. 291. Ood-rach. उदराच عودراچهه	Sapindus Emarginatus.	The seed and fruit given as emetic; and worn as a charm. Dose gr. i. to ℈ss. Price per lb. 0 3 8

Names, English and Country.	Botanical Names.	Remarks.
No. 292. Oonab. उनाब عُناب	Zisyphus Jujuba.	The dried imported jujubes: eaten as restorative. Dose ℥ss. to ℥ii. Price per lb. 0 8 0
No. 293. Peepla mor. पीपला मोर پیپلامور	Piper Longum.	The root of the long pepper; stimulating. Dose gr. v. to ℈i. Price per lb. 0 3 0
No. 294. Pockur-mool. पोखरमोखं پوکھرمول	Polygonum Hydropiper. (?)	The root is stimulating, bitter and tonic, and universally used as such. Dose ℈ss. to ʒss. Price per. lb 0 8 0
No. 295. Pattis. पाटइस پاتیس	Cyperus Inundatus.	The tubers are used as tonic and stimulating. Dose ℈i. to ʒi. Price per lb. 0 8 0

Names, English and Country.	Botanical Names.	Remarks.
No. 296. Pandrie. पांदरी پاندري	Bignonia Chelonoides.	The leaves used in infusion in cases of madness. Dose ℈i. to ʒii. in infusion. Price per lb. 2 8 0
No. 297. Padmuck. पादमक پدمکهه	Cerasus Caproniana.	The Cherry Tree of the Hills; the bark is used as astringent and febrifuge. Dose ℈ii. to ℥ss. Price per lb. 0 7 8
No. 298. Pakhun Bied. पाखनबेद پاکهان بید	Saxifraga Ciliosa.	The root used as tonic and bitter. Dose gr. v. to ℈i. Price per lb. 0 2 0
No. 299. Para. पारा پارا		Quicksilver, used both externally and internally, in combination many ways. Dose gr. ¼ to gr. ii. rubbed in ghee. Price per lb. 3 8 0

Names, English and Country.	Botanical Names.	Remarks.
No. 300. Pust-burn. पश्तबरन پست برن	Andropogon Nardus.	Spice grass. The leaves highly fragrant; used as stomachic. Dose ℈ss. to ʒii. in infusion. Price per lb. 5 0 0
No. 301. Papeeta. पापीता پپیته	Strychnos Scanti Ignatii.	St. Ignatius's Bean. The seed used as narcotic, stimulating and poisonous. Dose gr. $\frac{1}{6}$ to gr. iv. Price per lb. 0 8 0
No. 302. Phitkaree. फहटकीरी فیٹکري		Supersulphate of Alamina and Potash Alum. Used internally and externally. Dose gr. $\frac{1}{2}$ to gr. iv. Price per lb. 0 1 4
No. 303. Pukumbrie Nosadur. पकमबरी नोशादर پکهمبري نوسادر		Artificial Realgar; used by Fukeers to heat themselves within cold weather; by fumigation. Dose: not given internally. Price per lb. 2 0 0

Names, English and Country.	Botanical Names.	Remarks.
No. 304. Pharid-buti. फारीदबुटी فريدبوٹي	Cocculus Villosus. Menispermum Hirsutum.	Used as mucilaginous, the raw leaves and stems being rubbed up. The root considered heating, laxative, and sudorific. Dose gr. v. to ℈i. Price per lb. 0 1 0
No. 305. Palas pipul. Paris-ka-phull. पलाश पीपल پلاس پیپل	Hibiscus Populeoides.	Poplar Hibiscus. The seed used in horse medicines; and in purges. Dose gr. iii. to gr. ℈i. Price per lb. 0 3 8
No. 306. Padzehr. पादजेहर پادزهر		Bezoarstones used externally and internally in charm and medicines. Dose gr. ½ to gr. viii. Price per lb. 80 0 0
No. 307. Pahari pipul. पहारी पीपल پهاري پیپل	Piper Sylvaticum.	Wild Hill Pepper; used green and dried as condiment and carminative. Dose gr. v. to ℈i. Price per lb. 0 5 3

Names, English and Country.	Botanical Names.	Remarks.
No. 308. Post-bharoon pista. पोश्ततभेरून पइश्टा پوست بيرون پسته	Pistacia Vera.	The pericarp, resinous and used as stimulating and astringent. Dose gr. ii. to ℈i. Price per lb. 0 8 0
No. 309. Putcha-pat. पतचपाट پچاپات	Marrubium Odoratissimum.	Leaves imported from Singapore, and used in scents and tobacco. Dose: not given internally. Price per lb. 0 4 6
No. 310. Pista. पइश्ता پسته	Pistacia Vera.	Pistachio nuts, used as restorative. Dose ℥ss. to ʒii. Price per lb. 1 0 0
No. 311. Pia-ranga. पइआरंगा پيارانگا		The root imported from Arracan, used as an ingredient in many medicines; tonic. Dose gr. iii. to ℈i. Price per lb. 0 5 3

Names, English and Country.	Botanical Names.	Remarks.
No. 312. Patol. पाटोल پاتول	Trichosanthes Cordata.	Used as a bitter febrifuge and deobstruent. Dose gr. v. to ℈ii. Price per lb. 0 1 0
No. 313. Post-bekh-kibr. पोश्तबीचकइबर The Real Caper. پوست بیخ کبر	Capparis Spinosa.	The bark of the root used as expectorant and laxative. Dose gr. ii. to ℈ss. Price per lb. 0 7 6
No. 314. Paluk-juhi. पालकजुही پالک جوهي	Justicia Nasuta.	The root acrid and bitter and applied to cure herpes and ring worms. Dose: not given internally. Price per lb. 0 1 0
No. 315. Panyala. Talis-putrie. पानीआला پنیاله	Flacourtia Cataphracta.	The small leaves and shoots resemble rhubarb in flavour, and are used as gentle astringents. Dose ℈ii. to ℥ii. Price per lb. 0 2 0

Names, English and Country.	Botanical Names.	Remarks.
No. 316. Pammuhoorie. पानमऊरी پان‌مهوري	Fœniculum Panmorium.	The root used as an aromatic in food and medicine. Dose gr. x. to ℈ii. Price per lb. 1 8 0
No. 317. Phulsa. फलसा فلسا	Grewia Asiatica.	The fruit cooling, the bark astringent. Dose gr. v. to ʒss. Price per lb. 0 1 0
No. 318. Pumba-dana. पमबादाना پنبه‌دانه	Gossypium Herbaceum.	Seed; given as a stimulant. Dose ℈ss. to ℈ii. Price per lb. 0 1 0
No. 319. Pit-papra. पइतपापरा پیت‌پاپرا	Butea Frondosa.	The large flat seeds, used an anthelmentic and deobstruent. Dose gr. iii. to ℈i. Price per lb. 0 3 6

Names, English and Country.	Botanical Names.	Remarks.
No. 320. Putranjiva. पतरानजीवा پترنجیوه	Putranjiva Roxburghii.	The nuts are strung round the necks of children to keep them well. Dose: not given internally. Price per lb. 0 10 0
No. 321. Putruj. पतरज پترج	Laurus Malabathrum.	The bark used as cinnamon. Dose ℈ss. to ℈ii. Price per lb. 0 6 0
No. 322. Phurrud. फरद پهرهد	Erythrinum Corallodendron.	The bark is used as stimulant and tonic, and is very bitter. Dose ℈ii. to ʒi. in infusion. Price per lb. 0 1 0
No. 323. Rai. रै رائي	Sinapis Nigra and Dichotoma.	Several kinds of Mustard seed are much used, both internally and externally. Dose ʒss. to ʒii. Price per lb. 0 0 8

Names, English and Country.	Botanical Names.	Remarks.
No. 324. Ruskapoor. रसकापुर رس کپور		Impure protochloride of mercury; used as a purge, and in ointments. Dose gr. $\frac{1}{4}$ to gr. v. well washed in hot water. Price per lb. 6 4 0
No. 325. Roomie Mastungi. रुमीमसटगी رومي مستكي	Pistacia Lentiscus.	Mastich used as a perfume, also as an aphrodisiac. Dose gr. v. to ℈i. Price per lb. 1 4 6
No. 326. Rendhie. रैंधी رينڈي	Ricinius Communis.	Castor oil, used as a common purge. Dose ʒss. to ℥ii. Price per lb. 0 0 8
No. 327. Rewund Kutai. रेवंद काटै ريونه خطائي	Rheum Palmatum.	Rhubarb root, used as a purge and diuretic: also an extract. Dose gr. v. to ʒiss. Price per lb. 2 8 0

Names, English and Country.	Botanical Names.	Remarks.
No. 328. Rewund Chini. रेवंद चीनी ریوند چینی	Rumex Tuberosus.	A darber root like rhubarb, of an inferior kind. Dose ℈ss. to ʒii. Price per lb. 0 10 0
No. 329. Reg-Mahee. Lacertus Scincus. रेगमाही ریگ ماهي		The skink; imported from Cabul, and used as restorative and aphrodisiac—It is brought dried and varnished., Dose ʒi. to ʒii. Price per lb. 12 0 0
No. 330. Rahoosa-ka-tel. रऊस्रा का तेल رهوسا کا تیل	Andropogon Martini.	Roosa oil; used as a stimulant and rubefacient. Dose i. to viii. Price per lb. 19 0 0
No. 331. Ral. राल رال	Vatica Robusta. Shorea Robusta.	Rosin of two kinds; used externally and given to check hœmorrhage. Dose gr. ii. to ℈i. Price per lb. 0 0 8

Names, English and Country.	Botanical Names.	Remarks.
No. 332. Ram puttrie. रामपटरी رام پتري	Myristicha Macrophylla.	The dried arillus of this kind of nutmeg tree is quite tasteless and scentless and inert; given as aphrodisiac. Dose gr. ii. to ℈i. Price per lb. 2 8 0
No. 333. Resha-kutmie. रेशाखतमी Resha-kitmie. ريسه خطمي	Sida Mauritiana.	The root used as refrigerant and mucilaginous. Dose ℥ss. to ℥ii. in infusion. Price per lb. 0 5 4
No. 334. Rusawat. रशावत رسوت	Berberis Asiatica.	The extract of the Hill Berberry Wood; used externally and internally as discutient and deobstruent. Dose gr. v to ℈i. Price per lb. 0 10 0
No. 335. Ruchna. रचना رچنا		The root boiled in oil; used to rub the body with in rheumatism, also given in fever. Dose gr. ii. to ℈ss. Price per lb. 0 8 0

Names, English and Country.	Botanical Names.	Remarks.
No. 336. Rohunna. रोहना روهنا	Soymida Febrituga. Swictenia Febrifuga.	The bark used as a tonic. Dose ʒi. to ℥ss. in infusion. Price per lb. 0 0 8
No. 337. Rooman. रुमान رومان	Punica Granatum.	The bark of the root; used as deobstruent and applied externally; and given in tape worm. Dose gr. iii. to ℈i. Price per lb. 0 1 0
No. 338. Ruchta-Semul. रक्ताशेमल رکتاسینبل	Salmalia Malabrica. Bombax Heptaphyllum.	The dried flowers used as demulcent. Dose ʒii. to ℥i. in infusion. Price per lb. 0 0 8
No. 339. South. शोट سونٹهه	Zingiber Officinale.	Dried ginger, extensively used both internally and externally and in food. Dose gr. iii. to ʒss. Price per lb. 0 2 0

Names, English and Country.	Botanical Names.	Remarks.
No. 340. Siya-Jeera. शीयाजीरा سیاہ زیرہ	Carum Carui.	The seed used as carminative and stimulant. Dose gr. iii. to ʒss. Price per lb. 0 5 3
No. 341. Sohaga. शोहागा سوہاگہ		Bi-Borate of Soda, used extensively externally; also given internally as a laxative. Dose ℈i. to ʒii. Price per lb. 0 3 8
No. 342. Sutowar. Shutmoola. शटोवार ست مولا	Asparagus Racemosus.	The root is used as stimulant and restorative. Dose ʒi. to ℥ss. Price per lb. 0 2 0
No. 343. Sikakul. Shekakul. शीकाकुल سقاقل	Ænanthe crocata (?) Sium Ninsi.	Wild water parsnep used as an aphrodisiac. Dose gr. ii. to ℈ss. Price per lb. 0 4 0

Names, English and Country.	Botanical Names.	Remarks.
No. 344. Soorinjan. सुरइनजान سرنجان	Colchicum Illyricum. Hermodactylus. Colchicum Variegatum.	The Hermodactyl roots, used as cathartics, and also as aphrodisiacs. Dose gr. $\frac{1}{4}$ to gr. v. Price per lb. 1 4 0
No. 345. Sumoondur Sokh. समुनदर शोख سمندرسوکهه	Argyreia Speciosa. Lettsomia Trivervia.	The seed used with Salep Misre as an aphrodisiac; the half roasted leaves applied to the skin are escharotic. Dose gr. iii. to ℈i. Price per lb. 0 2 0
No. 346. Sumoondar-jug. Sumoondar phen. समुनदरजग سمندرجهگ		The bone of the cuttle fish; used as refrigerant; used in eye ointments. Dose gr. iii. to ʒss. Price per lb. 0 12 0
No. 347. Sehora. सीहोरा سیهورا	Trophis Aspera.	The bark is used as a tonic; and is supposed to charm away snakes. Dose gr. i. to ℈ss. Price per lb. 0 1 0

Names, English and Country.	Botanical Names.	Remarks.
No. 348. Sumundur-phull. समुनदरफल سمندرپهل	Barringtonia Acutangula.	The fruit is intoxicating; the root is used as aperient, cooling and febrifuge. Dose gr. iii. to ℈i. Price per lb. 0 0 8
No. 349. Soorma. सुरमा سرمه		Sulphuret of Antimony used extensively externally. Dose: not given internally. Price per lb. 0 8 0
No. 350. Soorma Sufaid. सुरमा सफेद سرمه سفيد		Carbonate of Lime. Double Refracting Spar. Used to the eyes, and also to clean the teeth. Dose: not given internally. Price per lb. 0 2 0
No. 351. Souf-ka-jur. सौंफ का जड़ سونف کا جڑ	Pimpinella Anisum.	The root used as carminative and deobstruent. Dose ℈ss. to ʒi. Price per lb. 0 1 0

Names, English and Country.	Botanical Names.	Remarks.
No. 352. Soa-ka-beej. सोया का बीज سویا کا بیج	Anethum Soa.	The seed used as carminative and digestive. Dose ℈ss. to ʒi. Price per lb. 0 1 0
No. 353. Sooriyalee. सुराली سورالي	Amaranthus Cernua.	The seed used as refrigerant and astringent. Dose ℈ss. to ʒii. Price per lb. 0 1 0
No. 354. Senna Mukhie. सनामखी سنامکي	Cassia Senna.	Senna Leaves; used as a common purge. Dose ʒss. to ℥i. in infusion. Price per lb. 0 4 0
No. 355. Salep Misrie. सालहपमहसरी ثالبمصري	Orchis Mascula.	The roots eaten as restorative and aphrodisiac. Dose ʒii. to ℥ii. Price per lb. 10 0 0

Names, English and Country.	Botanical Names.	Remarks.
No. 356. Satsarila. शटशरीला ست سریلا	Myrica Sapida.	The flowers of the Kaiphull tree, smell sweetly; used dry in messales; as restorative. Dose ʒss. to ʒii. Price per lb. 45 0 0
No. 357. Sung-turash. शंगतराश سنگ تراش		Steatite, used to polish stones and lime; also eaten by women in "luddoo;" called also "Paupak." Dose gr. iii. to ℈ii. Price per lb. 0 12 0
No. 358. Sisa. Boondee; Lead. शीशा سیسہ		The oxides given as aphrodisiacs and used in ointments. Dose gr. $\frac{1}{8}$ to gr. i. ss. Price per lb. 0 4 0
No. 359. Sumbhul Khar. Arsenic. शम्भलखार سنبل کھار		Arsenious Acid; used to cure leprosy, snake bites and other diseases; applied externally in ointments. Dose gr. $\frac{1}{60}$ Price per lb. 7 8 0

Names, English and Country.	Botanical Names.	Remarks.
No. 360. Sugandh mattrie. सुगंधमाटरी سوگندہ ماتري Gundho Malutee.	Echites Caryophyllata.	The root used in tobacco and in dyes on account of the scent. Dose gr. v. to ℈i. Price per lb. 0 2 6
No. 361. Sathara; Shaturrah. Pitpapra; Ufyloon. शाथारा شہترہ	Fumaria Parviflora.	The dried stalks and leaves used as a tonic and febrifuge. Dose ʒi. to ℥i. in infusion. Price per lb. 0 2 0
No. 362. Sanda. Sand. सांदा سانڈہ		A species of lizard, the oil of which is used as aphrodisiac. Dose: not given internally. Price per lb. 5 0 0
No. 363. Sugandh-kokla. सुगंधकोकला سوگندہ کوکلا	Xanthoxylum Budrunga. Fagara Budrunga.	Aromatic sweet scented berries; are used in making scents, and abound in oil and resins; as a refrigerant. Dose ℈ss. to ʒi. Price per lb. 0 3 0

Names, English and Country.	Botanical Names.	Remarks.
No. 364. Salburnie. Saloon. शालबरणी سال برني Salpan.	Desmodium Gangeticum.	The leaves and stalks considered stimulating. Dose ℈ii. to ℥i. in infusion. Price per lb. 10 0 0
No. 365. Sufaid chirmie. Sufaid Ghoonchie. सफेदघुंची سفيدگهونگچي	Abrus Precatorius.	The white kind are reckoned stimulating, also the red kind; "soorkh chirmie." Dose gr. ¼ to gr. ii. Price per lb. 0 5 3
No. 366. Suja-balud. Shah Ballat. शाहबालोट شاه بالوت	Quercus Gramuntia. Quercus Ballota.	The acorns are used as tonic and astringent. Dose ℈i. to ℥ss. Price per lb. 2 8 0
No. 367. Sung-sir-mahee. संगसीरमाही سنگسرماهي		A concretion from the head of a fish; used as an aphrodisiac. Dose grss. to ℈i. Price per lb. 5 0 0

Names, English and Country.	Botanical Names.	Remarks.
No. 368. Sung-Misrie. संगमइसरी سنگ مصري		The stone imported from Cabul; used as an aphrodisiac. Dose gr. ¼ to gr. i. Price per lb. 5 0 0
No. 369. Sutr-sowa. सटरसोवा ستر سويا Hub-ool-ass.	Myrtus Communis.	Myrtle berries and leaves used as carminative and refrigerant and in scents; and as astringents. Dose ℈ii. to ʒii. Price per lb. 2 8 0
No. 370. Sheerkist. शीरखइसत شيرخست	Fraxinus Florifera.	Ash mannca, used as a slight purge. Dose ℈i. to ℥iss. Price per lb. 11 4 0
No. 371. Sirka. शीरका سركه		Vinegar; the best at Patna is made from the juices of the Borassus Flabelli formis and Phœnix Dactylifera and Sylvestris. Refrigerant. Dose ʒii. to ℥iss. Price per lb. 0 0 8

Names, English and Country.	Botanical Names.	Remarks.
No. 372. Sowan-mukhie. Sona-mukhie. शोवानमषी سوانمكهي		Sulphuret of Iron. Iron pyrites; considered refrigerant and tonic; and used in itch ointments. Dose gr. ½ to ℈i. Price per lb. 2 8 0
No. 373. Sahut. शाहत شهت		Honey; much used in medicines. Dose ℈i. to ℥i. Price per lb. 0 2 8
No. 374. Sung-dirayo. शंगदरीयाउ سنگدريا		Impure nitro muriatic acid; used as cooling and astringent. Dose m. iii. to viii. Price per lb. 15 0 0
No. 375. Sung-jerahut. शंगजीराहत سنگ جراحت Surkoola. Sungderaz.		Used to unite wounds; a kind of steatite. Dose: not given internally. Price per lb. 0 2 0

Names, English and Country.	Botanical Names.	Remarks.
No. 376. Soogandh-bala. सुगंधबाला سوگندهبالا	Pavonia Odorata.	The scented roots infused as a diet drink in fevers. Dose ʒi. to. ℥ii. in infusion. Price per lb. 0 4 8
No. 377. Shistie. शस्शटी سیستي	Salvia Bengalensis.	The leaves are used in scents. Dose: not given internally. Price per lb. 0 1 0
No. 378. Surhunchee-ka-jur. शरहनची का जड़ سرهنچي کا جڑ	Alternanthera Sessilis.	The root stimulant; and used to apply to boils and abscesses. Dose: not given internally Price per lb. 0 1 0
No. 379. Shah-booi. शाहबुइ ساہبوئي		A kind of bark, used as a scent, and also as an aphrodisiac. Dose gr. i. to ℈ss. Price per lb. 5 0 0

Names, English and Country.	Botanical Names.	Remarks.
No. 380. Sheal-kanta. Bhut-kutaya. शीयकांटा سيال كانٹا	Argemone Mexicana.	Used to stimulate ulcers; the fresh juice being applied. Dose: not given internally. Price per lb. 0 0 3
No. 381. Saboon-Mittie. साबुनमट्टी سابونمٹي		Fullers Earth used in "luddoo" to check diarrhœa. Dose ℈i. to ʒi. Price per lb. 0 4 0
No. 382. Shukur-teghal. शकरतेघाल سکرتيغال		The nidus of an insect in repute in epilepsy. Dose gr. ii. to ℈ss. Price per lb. 2 8 0
No. 383. Saheba. साहीबा ساهيبا	Artemisia Judaica.	Indian Semen Contra; used as an anthelmintic—excessively bitter; tonic and stimulant. Dose gr. iii. to ʒss. Price per lb. 10 0 0

Names, English and Country.	Botanical Names.	Remarks.
No. 384. Sindoor. Minium सइनदूर سندور		Red lead; used in various ointments. Dose: not given internally. Price per lb. 0 3 0
No. 385. Subze-ke-beej सबजी की बीज سبزي کا بيج	Ocimum Sanctum.	Black Toolsee seed; demulcent and refrigerant. Dose ʒss. to ℥ss. Price per lb. 0 2 6
No. 386. Sad. साद سعد	Cyperus Triangularis.	Triangular leaved Mootha. The root used as tonic and as a scent. Dose ℈ss. to ʒi. Price per lb. 0 5 0
No. 387. Sadan. सावदान سعدان	Cyperus Geminatus.	The twin root used as diuretic and restorative. Dose ℈ss. to ʒi. Price per lb. 0 5 0

Names, English and Country.	Botanical Names.	Remarks.
No. 388. Suphadie-khuss. सफादीखस سفادیکس	Ledebouria Hyacinthina. Erythronium Indicum.	The roots used as narcotic and diuretic. Dose grss. to gr. iii. Price per lb. 2 8 0
No. 389. Suphur-jul. सफरजल سفرجل	Cydonia Vulgaris.	The quince fruit dried and sliced used in sherbets as refrigerant. Dose ℥ss. to ℥i. Price per lb. 1 8 0
No. 390. Siris-ka-beej. सिरिस का बीज سریس کا بیج	Mimosa Seris.	The seed used as astringent in diarrhœa. Dose ℈ss. to ʒss. Price per lb. 0 1 0
No. 391. Sookh. सुख سوکهه	Emblica Officinalis.	The dried juice of the anola; used as astringent, and as a condiment. Dose gr. v. to ℈i. Price per lb. 2 8 0

Names, English and Country.	Botanical Names.	Remarks.
No. 392. Silajeet. शइलाजीत سیلاجیت Storax.	Styrax Officinalis.	The gum resin used as fragrant and stimulating. Dose gr. ½ to ℈ss. Price per lb. 1 8 0
No. 393. Surhatta. शरहटा سرهٹا	Solanum Melongena.	The wild egg plant; the fruit given as febrifuge and tonic. Dose ℈i. to ʒi. in infusion. Price per lb. 0 1 0
No. 394. Sillarus. शीलारश سلارس Liquid Storax.	Liquid ambar Styraciflua.	Liquid Storax, used in scents, and as aphrodisiac. Dose gr. ii. to ℈i. Price per lb. 5 0 0
No. 395. Soomok. Shumac. शुमाक سوماق	Rhus Coriaria.	The leaves and bark and fruit used as refrigerant. Dose gr. ii. to ℥ss. Price per lb. 0 5 0

Names, English and Country.	Botanical Names.	Remarks.
No. 396. Sumsum. Til. समसम سمسم	Sesamum Orientale.	The seed used as demulcent; and eaten as food. Dose ʒii. to ℥ss. Price per lb. 0 0 8
No. 397. Sunkootun. सनकुटन سنكوتن	Smyphýtum Officinale.	The root is very mucilaginous and used to unite wounds. Dose not given internally. Price per lb. 0 8 0
No. 398. Sumbaduj. Kroon. समबादज سنبادج		A kind of stone of three different qualities; used as emery; given as tonic. Dose gr. ½ to ℈ss. Price per lb. 0 8 0
No. 399. Sembel-jibilee. सइमबइल जीबइली سنبل جيبلي	Valeriana Dioscoridis ?	A species of valerian used in scents and Sherbets. Dose ℈ss. to ℥i. Price per lb. 12 0 0

Names, English and Country.	Botanical Names.	Remarks.
No. 400. Sembel Roomie. सम्बल रूमी سنبل رومي	Valeriana Phu?	A similar root, used in scents and sherbets. Dose ℈ss. to ʒi. Price per lb. 12 0 0
No. 401. Sung Rassikh. संग रासिख سنگ راسخ		Impure black lead used in charms. Dose: not given internally. Price per lb. 10 0 0
No. 402. Sufaida. सफेदा سفیده		Impure Carbonate of Lead, used in ointments. Dose not given internally. Price per lb. 0 5 0
No. 403. Sutanuj. Sadnuj. सटानज صادنج Craw fish.		The concretions found in the stomach of the Cancer Astacus; used as application to piles. Dose: not given internally. Price per lb. 5 0 0

Names, English and Country.	Botanical Names.	Remarks.
No. 404. Suka-kool misrie. Shekakool misrie. शाकुल मइशरी سقاقل مصري	Daucus Sylvestris.	This kind is imported from Arabia and Egypt; and is used as a diuretic. Dose ʒss. to ʒii. in infusion. Price per lb. 2 8 0
No. 405. Sunk-choorun. शंकचूरन سنکهه چورن		Shavings of the conch shell; considered binding. Dose ℈i. to ʒi. Price per lb. 0 4 0
No. 406. Tuj तज تج	Laurus Nobilis.	The bark of the bay tree; used as cinnamon. Dose gr. ii. to ℈ss. Price per lb. 0 0 8
No. 407. Tal-Makhana. Kanta-Koolika. तालमखाना تال مکهانا	Asteracantha Longifolia. Ruellia Longifolia.	The seeds used as mucilaginous, tonic, and diuretic. Dose ℈ss. to ʒii. in infusion. Price per lb. 0 2 0

Names, English and Country.	Botanical Names.	Remarks.
No. 408. Tookhum Mullunga. तूखम मलंगा تخم ملنگا	Dracocephalum Royleanum.	The seeds are much used as mucilaginous. Dose ʒi. to ℥i. in infusion. Price per lb. 0 4 0
No. 409. Tej pata. तेजपाता تیج پتا	Laurus Malabathrum.	The leaves used as stimulant aromatics in food and medicine. Dose ʒss. to ʒi. Price per lb. 0 2 0
No. 410. Tugur. तगर تگر	Tabernœmontana Coronaria.	The wood used in incense, and as a scent, also in medicine, as refrigerant. Dose gr. iii. to ℈ss. Price per lb. 0 4 0

Names, English and Country.	Botanical Names.	Remarks.
No. 411. Treeak-pharook-roomia. तरयाकफारूकरुमी تریاق فاروق	Teucrium Chamœdrys.	An extract made from Teucrium Chamœdrys and other narcotic plants; the ancient Theriaca Andromachii; given in convulsions. Dose gr. ¼ to gr. v. Price per lb. 30 0 0
No. 412. Tookhum-kurpus. तुखमकरपस تخم کرفس	Apium Graveolens.	The seeds used as stimulant. Dose gr. iii. to ℈i. Price per lb. 0 8 0
No. 413. Tookhum-gundheena. तुखमगंदीना تخم گدینا	Allium Sativun.	Garlic seed used as diuretic. Dose ℈ss to ʒii. in infusion. Price per lb. 0 2 0
No. 414. Toorunj-been. तुरंजबीन ترنجبین	Hedysarum Alhugi. Alhugi Maurorum.	A kind of manna from this thorny plant; laxative. Dose ℈ii. to ℥ss. Price per lb. 1 4 0

Names, English and Country.	Botanical Names.	Remarks.
No. 415. Toombhool. तूमभूल تومل	Hypericum Patulum.	The scented seed used as an aromatic stimulant, comes from Nepal. Dose gr. ii. to ℈ss. Price per lb. 0 2 0
No. 416. Todrie-sufaid. तादरीश्रफेद تودري سفيد	Mathiola Longipetala.	The seed is used as aphrodisiac. Dose gr. v. to ʒss. Price per lb. 0 10 0
No. 417. Tookhm-gandha. तूखमगंधा تخم گنده	Alium Cepa.	Onion seed; used as diuretic. Dose gr. v. to ʒi. Price per lb. 0 2 0
No. 418. Tookhm-khutmai. तूखमखटमै تخم خطمي Great Hollyhock.	Althæa Rosea.	The seed and root used as mucilaginous. Dose ℈ to ℥ss. in infusion. Price per lb. 0 5 0

Names, English and Country.	Botanical Names.	Remarks.
No. 419. Tookhm-kahoo. तूखमकाहू تخم کاهو	Lactuca Sativa.	The seed used as mucilaginous. Dose ʒss. to ʒii. in infusion. Price per lb. 0 2 6
No. 420. Toormooz. तूरमुज ترمس	Lupinus Luteus.	The lupin pods are brought from Egypt, and used as carminative. Dose gr. ii. to ℈i. Price per lb. 2 8 0
No. 421. Tookhm-koolpha. तूखमकुलफा تخم قلفه	Portulaca Oleracea.	Common purslain; the seed used as demulcent and diuretic. Dose ʒi. to ʒii. in infusion. Price per lb. 0 2 6
No. 422. Todrie-soorookh. तोदरीसूरख تودري سرخ	Cheiranthus Cheiri.	Wall flower; the seed is used as aphrodisiac. Dose gr. v. to ℈i. Price per lb. 0 5 0

Names, English and Country.	Botanical Names.	Remarks.
No. 423. Thal-moolie. थालमुली تال‌مولي	Aponogeton Monostachyon.	The root is used as aphrodisiac and restorative. Dose ʒii. to ℥ss. Price per lb. 0 8 0
N.o 424. Thaikul. थैकल تهيكل	Hebadendron Pictorium.	A kind of gamboge from this tree, used as a purgative. Dose gr. ¼ to gr. vii. Price per lb. 1 4 0
No. 425. Thal-kesur. थालकेशर تال‌کيسر	Strychnos Nux Vomica.	The bark given as tonic, stimulant and narcotic, and as aphrodisiac. Dose gr. ⅛ to gr. ii. Price per lb. 0 4 0
No. 426. Tej-bul. तेजबल تيج‌بل	Xanthoxylum Hastile.	The bark used as astringent; and the seed and capsules narcotic, and used to intoxicate fish, also chewed as sialagogue. Dose gr. ii. to ℈i. Price per lb. 0 4 6

Names, English and Country.	Botanical Names.	Remarks.
No. 427. Telini. तेलीनी تیلیني	Meloe Cichorii. Meloe Trianthema.	Blistering fly; used to raise blisters. Dose: not given internally. Price per lb. 0 8 0
No. 428. Turbad. वरबाद تربد	Ipomœa Turpethum.	Turbeth root; used as cathartic. Dose gr. iii. ʒi. Price per lb. 0 2 0
No. 429. Thikoor. थइकूर تکهور	Curcuma Leucorrhiza.	A fine amylaceus farina, equal to arrow root is prepared from this root. Dose: used as food. Price per lb. 0 2 0
No. 430. Tisi. तइसी تیسي	Linum Usitatissimum.	Common flax; the seed used as demulcent. Dose ʒi. to ℥i. in infusion. Price per lb. 0 0 8

Names, English and Country.	Botanical Names.	Remarks.
No. 431. Titaliya. तीताळीया تیتولیا	Sonchus Ciliatus.	Sow thistle. The leaves and root used as tonic and febrifuge. Dose ʒii. to ℥ii. in infusion. Price per lb. 0 0 8
No. 432. Unjeera. Unjeeroot. आनजीरा انجیرہ	Penœa Sarcocolla.	Sarcocolla supposed to heal wounds rapidly. Dose: applied externally. Price per lb. 1 4 0
No. 433. Us-abai-hoormuz. आभ्राबैह्लरमज عسابۂهرمس	Colchicum Illyricum.	The flowers of the hermodactyl plant; used as cathartic. Dose gr. iv. to ℈i. in infusion. Price per lb. 17 0 0
No. 434. Unjeer. आनजीर انجیر	Ficus Carica.	Figs; much used as restorative. Dose; eaten as food. Price per lb 0 10 0

Names, English and Country.	Botanical Names.	Remarks.
No. 435. Ununta-mool. आनंतामुल اننتمول	Hemidesmus Indicus.	The root used as an excellent tonic. Dose ʒii. to ℥iss. in decoction. Price per lb. 1 10 0
No. 436. Urzoon. Arjun. आरजुन ارجُن	Terminalia Alata.	The fruit used as tonic and deobstruent. Dose gr. v. to ℈ii. Price per lb. 0 4 6
No. 437. Usluk. आस्लक اسلکهه	Vitex Agnus Castus.	The chaste tree. The seed is used by this native name as stimulant and aphrodisiac. Dose gr. viii. to ʒss. Price per lb. 5 0 0
No. 438. Ur-shud. आरशहद ارشد		The marcasite stone, used as heating and tonic. Dose gr. ¼ to gr. vi. Price per lb. 5 0 0

Names, English and Country.	Botanical Names.	Remarks.
No. 439. Us-koo-roon. आसकूरून اسکورن		Subcarbonate of iron; given as a tonic. Dose gr. ii. to ℈i. Price per lb. 0 2 0
No. 440. Ukhoond. आखुंद اکوند	Calotropis Odorifera.	The root bark is used like mudar but is weaker. Dose gr. iss. to ʒi. Price per lb. 0 1 0
No. 441. Usul-ool-nilofar. आसलउलनीलोफर اصل النيلوفر	Nymphœa Lotus.	The root used as restorative. Dose; eaten as food in milk. Price per lb. 0 8 0
No. 442. Utees. आटीस اتیس	Asparagus Sarmentosus.	The root used as restorative and tonic. Dose; ʒii. to ℥i. Price per lb. 0 5 3

Names, English and Country.	Botanical Names.	Remarks.
No. 443. Udhie-charie. अधीचारी ادهيچاره	Achyranthes Aspera.	The dried spikes are given in hydrophobia. Dose; ʒss. to ʒi. in infusion. Price per lb. 0 0 6
No. 444. Am-ka-gootlee. आम का गुटली ام كي گوتهلي	Mangifera Indica.	The seed used as febrifuge. Dose; gr. ii. to ℈i. Price per lb. 0 0 6
No. 445. Unfak. आनफाक انفاق	Olea Europœa.	The oil used as rubefacient. Imported from Persia. Dose: not given internally. Price per lb. 5 0 0
No. 446. Surphonka. शरफोका سرپهونكا	Galega Purpurea.	The plant used as tonic and febrifuge. Dose ʒii. to ℥ii. in infusion Price per lb. 0 1 6

Names, English and Country.	Botanical Names.	Remarks.
No. 447. Sokh. शोख سوکهه Asokh.	Uvaria Longifolia.	The wood used in fevers. Dose ℥ss. to ℥ii. in decoction. Price per lb. 0 0 6
No. 448. Umbul-dub. आमबलदब عنبرالدب	Solanum Œthiopicum.	The seeds given in asthma, and diarrhœa. Dose gr. ¼ to gr. iii. Price per lb. 2 8 0
No. 449. Unnum. Gool-anar. अनम گلِ انار	Punica Granatum.	The flowers of the double variety used as cooling and astringent. Dose ʒii. to ℥i. in infusion. Price per lb. 0 3 0
No. 450. Arusuk. Beer-bahootee. आरशक عرسک बीरबहूटी بيربهوٹي	Aranea Coccinea.	The scarlet spider, used as an external application in Herpes Circinatus. Dose: not given internally. Price per lb. 0 14 0

Names, English and Country.	Botanical Names.	Remarks.
No. 451. Kuhaila. कहैला کہلا		The bark is used in embrocations, and as aphrodisiac, and as astringent and stimulant. Dose gr. iii. to ℈ss. Price per lb. 0 5 0
No. 452. Uggur. आगर اگر	Aquillaria Agallocha.	Aloes' wood; used in scents and taken internally as refrigerant. Dose ℈ss. to ʒi. Price per lb. 2 8 0
No. 453. Umul-bet. Umbuti. आमलबेट املبیت	Oxalis Corniculata.	Procumbent sorrel. The stalks used as refrigerant and in condiments. Dose ℈ss. to ʒiss. Price per lb. 0 3 0
No. 454. Uzul-ool. आयुलउल انجلول Mazrioon. مازریون	Daphne Mazereon.	The root brought from Persia, and used as a stimulant sudorific. Dose ℈i. to ʒii. in decoction. Price per lb. 12 0 0

Names, English and Country.	Botanical Names.	Remarks.
No. 455. Zerawund. जहरावंद زراوند	Aristolochia Longa and Rotunda.	The roots bitter narcotic and stimulant; and used in snake bites. Dose gr. v. to ℈ii. Price per lb. 5 0 0
No. 456. Bala. बाला بالا	Paritium Tortuosum. Hibiscus Tortuosus.	The root given as febrifuge; and used in embrocations. Dose ℈i. to ʒii. Price per lb. 0 3 0
No. 457. Than. थान تهان	Althœa Rosea.	The root used as mucilaginous. Dose ʒii. to ℥i. in infusion. Price per lb. 0 1 0
No. 458. Rainoka. रैनोका رینوکا		The fruit, a small berry, used as tonic and febrifuge; and in embrocations. Dose gr. v. to ℈ii. Price per lb. 0 8 6

Names, English and Country.	Botanical Names.	Remarks.
No. 459. Bhedaira. भेदरौ بيدهاره	Gmelina Asiatica.	The root is used as mucilaginous, demulcent and restorative. Dose ʒii. to ℥ii. in infusion. Price per lb. 0 1 0
No. 460. Kurkurra. Ukul-kur. करकरा کرکرا	Canna Indica.	The root given in fevers by the poor; is demulcent. Dose ʒi. to ℥ss. in decoction. Price per lb. 0 1 0
No. 461. Kuniyala. कनीयला کنیالا		The root given as a laxative and as a stimulant. Dose ℈ss. to ℈ii. Price per lb. 0 8 0
No. 462. Kunkol. कंकोल کنکول		The fruit used as an aphrodisiac. Dose gr. v. to ℈i. Price per lb. 0 0 8

Names, English and Country.	Botanical Names.	Remarks.
No. 463. Tookhm-ferunjmishk. तुखमफइरइजमीश्क تخم فرنج مشک	Dracocephalum Moldavicum.	The seed used ground up in fevers and as demulcent. Dose ʒii. to ℥ss. in infusion. Price per lb. 0 10 0
No. 464. Cheer-kunkol. चीरकंकोल چهیرکنکول		The fruit is used as aphrodisiac and stimulant. Dose gr. v. to ℈i. Price per lb. 0 10 0
No. 465. Putal-kaura. पटालकौढ़ा پتال کونهره		The roots are given as stimulant and aphrodisiac. Dose ℈i. to ʒi. Price per lb. 1 4 6
No. 466. Buriara. बरोआरा بریارا	Sida Rhomboidæa.	The whole plant highly mucilaginous and used in dysentries. Dose ʒii. to ℥ii. in decoction. Price per lb. 0 0 6

Names, English and Country.	Botanical Names.	Remarks.
No. 467. Bundal. बंदाल بندال Sonekesur.	Vitis Carnosa.	The seeds used in embrocations; also the roots. Dose: not given internally. Price per lb. 0 0 8
No. 468. Kuhailee. काहेली كهيلي		The leaves and pods used as astringent and tonic. Dose gr. v. to ℈i. Price per lb. 0 2 0
No. 469. Juhazie-jaiphull. जहाजीजैफल جهاجي جايهل Jouz-jaiphull. جوزجايفل	Myristica Maccrocarpa.	The seed used as stimulant. Dose gr. v. to ℈ii. Price per lb. 5 0 6
No. 470. Rengnie. Khat-khataya. रेंगनी ريگني	Solanum Jacquini.	The root is given in decoction to cure fevers. Dose ʒi. to ʒii. in decoction. Price per lb. 0 0 6

Names, English and Country.	Botanical Names.	Remarks.
No. 471. Kurial. करीयाल كريال		The root is stimulant and used in embrocations. Dose: not given internally. Price per lb. 0 10 0
No. 472. Kuloonjie. Mugrela. कलोवनजी منگريلا	Nigella Indica.	The seed used as carminative; and applied externally. Dose gr. v. to ℈i. Price per lb. 0 0 8
No. 473. Bier-ke-gootie. बहर की गुटी بيرکا گوٹهي	Zisyphus Jujuba.	The seed used as astringent in diarrhœa. Dose ℈ii. to ʒii. Price per lb. 0 0 6
No. 474. Halim. हालहम هالم	Lepidium Sativum.	Common cress seed, used as stimulant and carminative. Dose gr. v. to ℈ii. Price per lb. 0 2 6

Names, English and Country.	Botanical Names.	Remarks.
No. 475. Tesu-ka-phool. तेसु का फुल تیسو کا پھول	Butea Frondosa.	The dried flowers used in dysmenorrhœa. Dose ℈ii. to ʒii. Price per lb. 0 2 0
No. 476. Buroon. बरुन برون	Cratœva Tapia.	The fruit and bark used in embrocations in rheumatism. Dose: not given internally. Price per lb. 0 1 0
No. 477. Bukchie. Babchee; Bapchie. बकची بکچی	Vernonia Anthelmintica. Conyza Anthelmintica. Serratula Anthelmintica.	The seeds are used pounded as an anthelmintic. Dose gr. v. to ℈ii. Price per lb. 0 1 0
No. 478. Chucka. चुका چکا	Croton Oblongifolium.	The fruit used as a purgative. Dose gr. ⅛ to gr. iii. Price per lb. 1 0 0

Names, English and Country.	Botanical Names.	Remarks.
No. 479. Gooma. گوما गुमा	Leonurus Tataricus.	The root, leaves and juice bitter ; used as febrifuge. Dose ʒii. to ℥ii. in infusion. Price per lb. 0 1 0
No. 480. Hutta-joorie. हाटाजुरी هتهاجوري Hutta-soora.	Heliotropium Indicum	The leaves used in fevers. Dose ʒss. to ʒiii. in infusion. Price per lb. 0 0 8

R. H. IRVINE, M. D.,
Civil Surgeon.

Patna, November 18*th*, 1847.

FINIS.